Executive Summary

Sexual, reproductive, maternal, newborn and adolescent health (SRMNAH) is an essential component of the Sustainable Development Goals (SDGs). Improving SRMNAH requires increased commitment to, and investment in, the health workforce. This report focuses primarily on midwives because they play a pivotal role within the wider SRMNAH workforce.

Following the universality principle of the SDGs, *State of the World's Midwifery 2021* (SoWMy 2021) represents an unprecedented effort to document the whole world's SRMNAH workforce. This approach acknowledges that not only low-income countries struggle to meet needs and expectations, especially in these difficult times, and that there are many paths to better SRMNAH: examples of good practice can be found in all countries, and all countries should be held to account.

The development and launch of SoWMy 2021 was led by the United Nations Population Fund (UNFPA) in partnership with the World Health Organization (WHO) and the International Confederation of Midwives (ICM), with the support of 32 organizations. It builds on previous reports in the SoWMy series in 2011 and 2014, and includes many countries not previously tracked.

The global SRMNAH worker shortage

In many countries, workforce planning and assessment of the workforce's ability to meet the need for health-care services is hampered by poor health workforce data systems. Based on the available data, SoWMy 2021 estimates that, with its current composition and distribution, the world's SRMNAH workforce could meet 75% of the world's need for essential SRMNAH care. However, in low-income countries, the workforce could meet only 41% of the need. Potential to meet the need is lowest in the African and Eastern Mediterranean WHO regions.

The SoWMy 2021 analysis indicates a current global needs-based shortage of 1.1 million "dedicated SRMNAH equivalent" (DSE) workers. There are shortages of all types of SRMNAH workers, but the largest shortage (900,000) is of midwives and the wider midwifery workforce. Investment is urgently needed to address this shortage.

At current rates, the SRMNAH workforce is projected to be capable of meeting 82% of the need by 2030: only a small improvement on the current 75%. The gap between low-income countries and high- and middle-income countries is projected to widen by 2030, increasing inequality.

To close the gap by 2030, 1.3 million new DSE worker posts (mostly midwives and mostly in Africa) need to be created in the next 10 years.

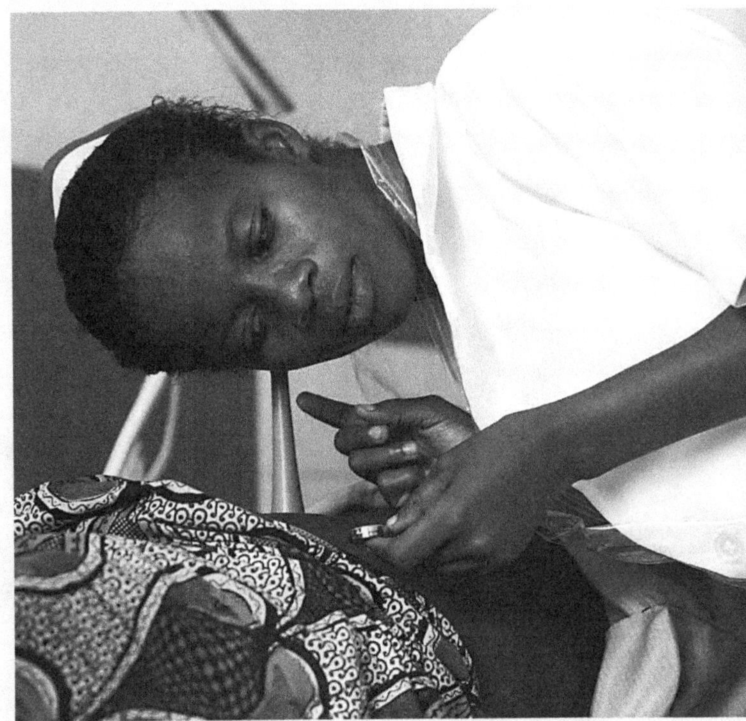

Lucia Sumani, a student midwife stationed at Balaka District Hospital, Malawi, conducts an antenatal check.
© Bill & Melinda Gates Foundation/Paul O'Driscoll.

At current rates, only 0.3 million of these are expected to be created, leaving a projected shortage of 1 million DSE posts by 2030, of which 750,000 will be midwives..

In addition to these shortages, the evidence points to the need to invest in improving quality of care and reducing the incidence of disrespect and abuse towards SRMNAH service users.

Why invest in midwives?

Since the first SoWMy report in 2011, the body of evidence demonstrating the return on investment in midwives has grown. It indicates that investing in midwives facilitates positive birth experiences and safe and effective comprehensive abortion services, improves health outcomes, augments labour supply, favours inclusive and equitable growth, facilitates economic stabilization, and can have a positive macroeconomic impact.

The Covid-19 pandemic has shone a light on the importance of investing in primary health care for meeting population health needs. Midwives are essential providers of primary health care and can play a major role in this area as well as other levels of the health system: in addition to maternity care, they provide a wide range of clinical interventions and contribute to broader health goals, such as addressing sexual and reproductive rights, promoting self-care interventions and empowering women and adolescent girls.

The analysis in this report indicates that fully educated, licensed and integrated midwives supported by interdisciplinary teams and an enabling environment can deliver about 90% of essential SRMNAH interventions across the life course, yet they account for less than 10% of the global SRMNAH workforce.

Bold investments are needed

For midwives to achieve their potential, greater investment is needed in four key areas: education and training; health workforce planning, management and regulation and the work environment; leadership and governance; and service delivery. Figure 1 provides a summary of the investments needed in each of these areas.

These investments should be considered at country, regional and global levels by

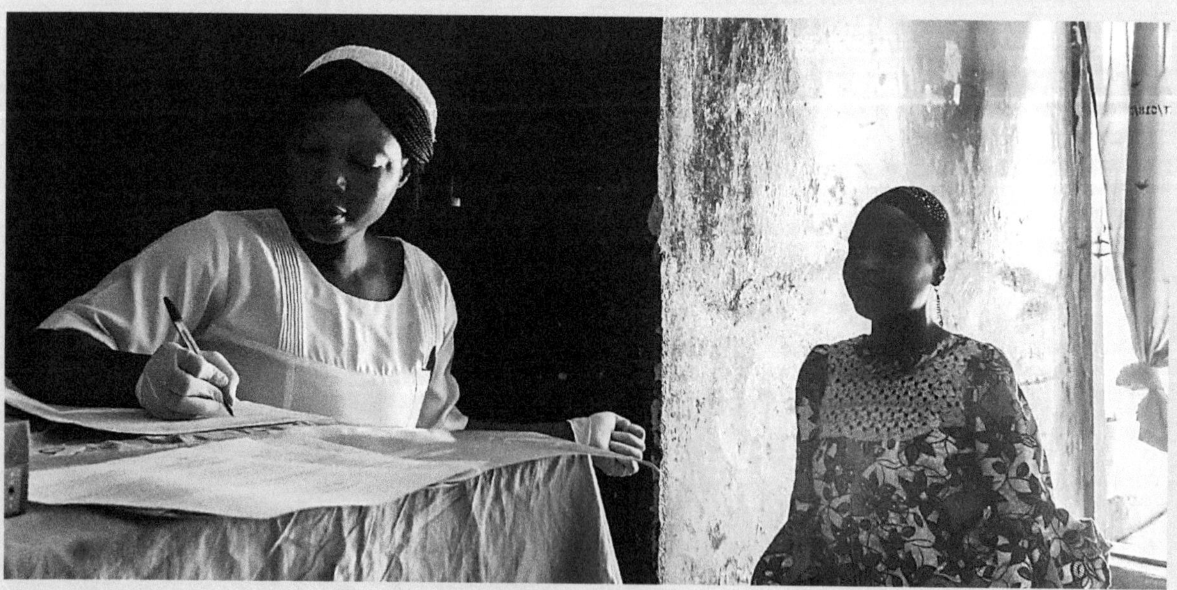

A midwife performs an antenatal check at the Primary Health Care Centre in Akwanga, Nasarawa State, Nigeria.
© Gates Archive/Nelson Owoicho.

Contents

BOXES

TABLES

FIGURES

Foreword

The Covid-19 crisis has prompted changes in how we think about health care and support: when and where it should be delivered, who should be involved, and what human and other resources should be prioritized. One important lesson is that even the most robust health systems can suddenly become fragile. We have seen during the crisis that women and girls have been affected in many ways, including increased gender-based violence and reduced access to essential sexual and reproductive health services, leading to increases in maternal mortality, unintended pregnancies, unsafe abortions and infant mortality.

Much of the evidence and analysis underpinning the *State of the World's Midwifery 2021* refers to the pre-Covid-19 era. The positive impact of high-quality midwifery care on women and families across the globe is richly detailed. The findings demonstrate the importance and effectiveness of midwives as core members of the sexual, reproductive, maternal, newborn and adolescent health (SRMNAH) workforce. They have been instrumental in helping to drive tangible progress towards several goals and targets of the 2030 Agenda for Sustainable Development.

In the face of Covid-19-related restrictions and overburdened health systems, midwives have become even more vital for meeting the sexual and reproductive health needs of women and adolescents. Midwives deserve to be celebrated for their courageous and often dangerous work during the crisis, which has helped to reduce the risk of virus transmission among pregnant women and their infants by enabling many births away from hospitals, either at home or in a midwifery unit or birth centre. Giving birth safely, comfortably and conveniently at home or in specialized community midwifery clinics is likely to be an increasingly popular option for pregnant women and their families in much of the world. Policy-makers are increasingly recognizing the overall efficiencies to be gained from investing in midwives and the infrastructure that sustains and supports them.

Governments and their partners should use the *State of the World's Midwifery 2021* to guide them on how and where attention and resources should be allocated to make this possible. The report reveals a global need for the equivalent of 1.1 million more full-time SRMNAH workers, mostly midwives and mostly in Africa. It also says that all countries need to improve the education and deployment of these occupation groups to meet demand by 2030. Decisions should also be informed by other important research findings, such as the fact that when fully educated, licensed and integrated in an interdisciplinary team, midwives can meet about 90% of the need for essential SRMNAH interventions across the life course. Currently, however, midwives comprise just 8% of the global SRMNAH workforce. Boosting that percentage, as well as the overall number of midwives, could be transformative. Universal coverage of midwife-delivered interventions could avert two thirds of maternal and neonatal deaths and stillbirths, allowing 4.3 million lives to be saved annually by 2035.

There is no better incentive to make midwives more central to all health systems and to ensure that they are educated, protected and treated as the valued professionals they are.

Deputy Secretary-General of the United Nations

governments, policy-makers, regulatory authorities, education institutions, professional associations, international organizations, global partnerships, donor agencies, civil society organizations and researchers.

The need to invest in the production and deployment of SRMNAH workers is not confined to countries with a needs-based shortage. Many countries, including some high-income countries, are forecast to have insufficient SRMNAH workers to meet demand by 2030.

The need for midwives and the wider SRMNAH workforce

Globally, 6.5 billion SRMNAH worker hours would have been required to meet all the need for essential SRMNAH care in 2019. This is projected to increase to 6.8 billion hours by 2030. Just over half (55%) of the need is for maternal and newborn health interventions (antenatal, childbirth and postnatal care), 37% is for other sexual and reproductive health interventions such as counselling, contraceptive services, comprehensive abortion care, and detection and management of sexually transmitted infections, and 8% is for adolescent sexual and reproductive health interventions.

Factors preventing the SRMNAH workforce from meeting all of the need include: insufficient numbers, inefficient skill mix, inequitable distribution, varying levels and quality of education and training programmes, limited qualified educators (including for supervision and mentoring) and limited effective regulation.

Covid-19 has reduced workforce availability. Access to SRMNAH services needs to be prioritized, and provided in a safe environment, despite the pandemic. SRMNAH workers need protection from infection, support to cope with stress and trauma, and creative/innovative solutions to the challenges of providing high-quality education and services.

Figure 1 **Summary of investments needed to enable midwives to achieve their potential**

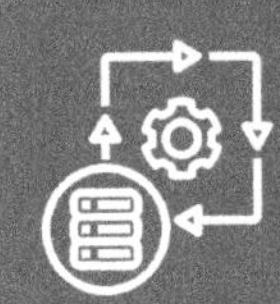

Health workforce data systems

Health workforce planning approaches that reflect the autonomy and professional scope of midwives

Primary health care, especially in underserved areas

Enabling and gender-transformative work environments

Effective regulatory systems

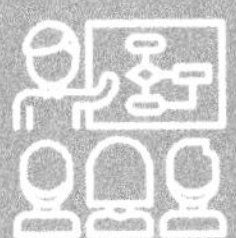

Educators and trainers

Education and training institutions

Communications and partnerships

Midwife-led models of care

Optimized roles for midwives

Applying the lessons from Covid-19

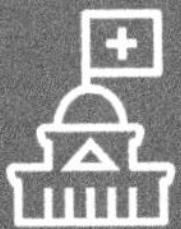

Creating senior midwife positions

Strengthening institutional capacity for midwives to drive health policy advancements

Equity of access to the SRMNAH workforce

Even where workforce data are available, they are rarely fully disaggregated by important characteristics such as gender, occupation group and geographical location, making it difficult to identify and address gaps in service provision.

Some population groups risk their access to SRMNAH workers being restricted due to characteristics including age, poverty, geographical location, disability, ethnicity, conflict, sexual orientation, gender identity and religion. The voices of service users are essential for understanding the factors that influence their care-seeking behaviour.

"Left behind" groups require special attention to ensure that they can access care from qualified practitioners. The SRMNAH workforce requires a supportive policy and working environment, and education and training, to understand and meet the specific needs of these groups and thus provide quality care that is accessible and acceptable to all.

Enabling and empowering the SRMNAH workforce

The health workforce is on average 70% women, with gender differences by occupation. Midwives are more likely to be women; they experience considerable gendered disparities in pay rates, career pathways and decision-making power.

Only half of reporting countries have midwife leaders within their national Ministry of Health. Limited opportunities for midwives to hold leadership positions and the scarcity of women who are role models in leadership positions hinder midwives' career advancement and their ability to work to their full potential.

Access to decent work that is free from stigma, violence and discrimination is essential to address gender-related barriers and challenges. All countries need policies to prevent attacks on health workers.

A gender transformative policy environment will challenge the underlying causes of gender inequities, guarantee the human rights, agency and well-being of caregivers, both paid and unpaid, recognize the value of health work and of women's work, and reward adequately.

*****

SoWMy 2021 was prepared during the world's struggle with Covid-19. We gratefully acknowledge the significant efforts made by stakeholders in many countries to provide data in the face of competing priorities, but it is clear that health workforce data systems were a major limitation even before the pandemic. Nevertheless, this report provides valuable new evidence to inform workforce policy and planning.

Since the first SoWMy report in 2011, there has been much progress in midwifery, including greater recognition of the importance of quality of care, widespread accreditation systems for health worker education institutions, and greater recognition of midwifery as a distinct profession. On the other hand, many of the issues highlighted in the two previous SoWMy reports remain of concern, such as workforce shortages, an inadequate working environment, low-quality education and training, and limitations in health workforce data.

Governments and relevant stakeholders are urged to use SoWMy 2021 to inform their efforts to build back better and fairer from the pandemic, forging stronger primary health-care systems as a pathway to UHC and fostering a more equitable world for all. It is hoped that the pandemic will be a catalyst for change given the heightened profile of health workers. SoWMy 2021 can help make this happen.

INTRODUCTION

Intense national efforts, supported by a number of global partnerships, have led to great progress over the past two decades in reducing maternal and newborn mortality and improving the health and well-being of women,[1] newborns and adolescents *(1)*. But progress has been uneven and too many are still being left behind. Global estimates point to approximately 810 maternal deaths every day *(2)*, one stillbirth every 16 seconds *(3)* and 2.4 million newborn deaths each year *(4)*, while almost one in five women gives birth without assistance from a skilled health provider *(5)*. An estimated 218 million women globally have unmet needs for modern contraception *(6)* and at least 10 million unintended pregnancies occur each year among 15–19-year-olds in low- and middle-income countries *(7)*. Emerging data from 2020 are starting to reveal the devastating effects of Covid-19 across these and other key indicators of sexual, reproductive, maternal, newborn and adolescent health (SRMNAH) *(8)*. The response to and recovery from the pandemic must prioritize meeting the SRMNAH needs of women, newborns, children, adolescents and families.

The "survive, thrive and transform" objectives of the United Nations (UN) Secretary-General's *Global Strategy for Women's, Children's and Adolescents' Health (2016–2030) (9)* aim, not only to reduce preventable deaths, but also to transform societies so that women, children and adolescents everywhere can realize their rights to the highest attainable standards of health and well-being. SRMNAH is an essential component of the Sustainable Development Goals (SDGs), particularly SDG 3: to "ensure healthy lives and promote well-being for all at all ages" and SDG 5: to "achieve gender equality and empower women and girls" *(10)*. Both the Global Strategy and the SDGs have at their core the imperatives to "leave no one behind" and to "reach the furthest behind first" *(11)*.

Resilient health systems grounded in primary health care are vital to the health and well-being of every woman, newborn and adolescent. The *Global Strategy on Human Resources for Health* stresses that without an effective health workforce no health system is viable and universal health coverage (UHC) cannot be achieved *(12)*. High-quality

> ⊙⇨ **KEY MESSAGES**
>
> ▶ Sexual, reproductive, maternal, newborn and adolescent health (SRMNAH) is an essential component of the Sustainable Development Goals. Improving SRMNAH requires increased commitment to, and investment in, the health workforce.
>
> ▶ This report focuses primarily on midwives because they play a pivotal role within the wider SRMNAH workforce. They can deliver most essential SRMNAH interventions across the life course if they are able to operate within a fully enabled health system and work environment.
>
> ▶ Building on reports in 2011 and 2014, the *State of the World's Midwifery 2021* (SoWMy 2021) represents an unprecedented effort to document the whole world's SRMNAH workforce and includes many countries not previously tracked.
>
> ▶ The devastating effects of Covid-19 are highlighted throughout this report. Governments and relevant stakeholders are urged to use SoWMy 2021 to inform their efforts to build back better and fairer from the pandemic.

---

1 SoWMy recognizes that individuals have diverse gender identities. Terms such as "pregnant person", "childbearing people" and "parent" can be used to avoid gendering those who give birth as feminine. However, because women are also marginalized and oppressed in most places around the world, we have continued to use the terms "woman", "mother" and "maternity". Our use of these words is not intended to exclude those who give birth and do not identify as women.

SRMNAH care requires a competent, educated, motivated and well supported workforce.

The *State of the World's Midwifery 2014* report (SoWMy 2014) and the subsequent regional and national reports (Box 1.1) led to some substantial advances, political commitments and achievements in a number of countries *(13)*. However, more needs to be done as a matter of urgency: SDGs 3 and 5 will not be met by 2030 without increased commitment to and investment in the education, recruitment, deployment, retention and management of midwives and other SRMNAH workers.

SoWMy 2021 was prepared during the world's struggle with Covid-19. Data collection and validation were severely hampered by health ministries' need to focus on responding to the pandemic. We gratefully acknowledge the significant efforts made by stakeholders in many countries to provide data in the face of competing priorities, but it is clear that health workforce data systems were a major limitation even before the pandemic. Nevertheless, this report provides valuable new evidence to inform workforce policy and planning.

Following the universality principle of the SDGs, SoWMy 2021 represents an unprecedented effort to document the whole world's SRMNAH workforce and therefore it includes many countries not previously tracked. This new approach acknowledges that not only low-income countries struggle to meet needs and expectations, especially in these difficult times, and that there are many paths to better SRMNAH: examples of good practice can be found in all countries, and all countries should be held to account.

The SRMNAH workforce and the central role of midwives

This report focuses primarily on midwives, but to understand their pivotal role it is necessary also to define and consider their place within the SRMNAH workforce. SoWMy 2021 uses international definitions to enable comparison across regions and countries and the International Standard Classification of Occupations (ISCO) system to classify the SRMNAH workforce into occupation groups based on their roles and responsibilities *(14)* (Table 1.1). Not all these occupations exist in every country, but where they do exist, and where data are available, they are included in the analysis. Definitions of each group can be found in Webappendix 1. The shaded groups in Table 1.1 indicate groups considered to be part of the "wider midwifery workforce" in this report.

Midwives' association

Previous *State of the World's Midwifery* reports

The first SoWMy report, *Delivering Health, Saving Lives (23)*, was launched at ICM's Triennial Congress in 2011. It was a response to the Global Call to Action issued at the Symposium on Strengthening Midwifery at Women Deliver in 2010 and aligned midwifery with the *Global Strategy for Women's and Children's Health*. The report provided a comprehensive analysis of midwifery services, education, regulation, deployment and conditions of service in 58 countries with high levels of maternal and newborn mortality.

The second report, *A Universal Pathway. A Woman's Right to Health (24)*, provided an evidence-base and detailed analysis of progress towards and challenges involved in delivering effective coverage of high-quality midwifery services in the 73 countries that collectively represented more than 95% of the global burden of maternal, newborn and child deaths. Launched at ICM's 30th Triennial Congress in 2014, the report has proved to be a valuable advocacy and evidence tool *(13)*.

There have also been four regional SoWMy reports *(25-28)* and several individual countries have conducted their own workforce assessments.

As in previous SoWMy reports, traditional birth attendants are not included because, although they attend a significant proportion of births in some countries and can play a role in community engagement and support *(15)*, many are not formally educated, trained or regulated. Community health workers, however, are included for the first time in a SoWMy report. Although they are variously defined and have differing competencies, they play an important role in many countries in delivering a small number of essential SRMNAH interventions. It is important to note that professionally qualified community midwives and nurses are distinct from community health workers.

About this report

The United Nations Population Fund (UNFPA) led the development and launch of SoWMy 2021 in partnership with the World Health Organization (WHO) and the International Confederation of Midwives (ICM), with the support of

TABLE 1.1

Occupation groups considered to be part of the SRMNAH workforce*

OCCUPATION GROUP	ISCO CODE	EXAMPLES
Midwifery professionals	2222	Professional midwife, technical midwife, midwife
Nursing professionals with midwifery training	2221	Nurse-midwife, perinatal nurse, maternity nurse
Nursing professionals	2221	Clinical nurse consultant, district nurse, nurse anaesthetist, nurse practitioner, operating theatre nurse, professional nurse, public health nurse, specialist nurse
Midwifery associate professionals	3222	Assistant midwife, auxiliary midwife
Nursing associate professionals with midwifery training	3221	Auxiliary nurse-midwife
Nursing associate professionals	3221	Assistant nurse, associate professional nurse, enrolled nurse, practical nurse, auxiliary nurse
Obstetricians and gynaecologists	2212	Obstetrician, gynaecologist
Paediatrician practitioners	2212	Paediatrician
General medical practitioners	2211	Family medical practitioner, general practitioner, medical doctor (general), medical officer (general), physician (general), primary care physician
Paramedical practitioners	2240	Advanced care paramedic, clinical officer (paramedical), feldscher, primary care paramedic, surgical technician, MEDEX
Medical assistants	3256	Clinical assistant, medical assistant
Community health workers	3253	Community health aide, community health promoter, community health worker, village health worker

* This list is not comprehensive; other SRMNAH occupation groups include dieticians and nutritionists, anaesthetists, pharmacists and physiotherapists. However, these groups (a) are considered necessary for the delivery of the essential SRMNAH interventions listed in the *Global Strategy for Women's, Children's and Adolescents' Health,* and (b) are identified in WHO's National Health Workforce Accounts platform.

Source: adapted from the International Labour Organization's International Standard Classification of Occupations ISCO-08 (14).

33 organizations. Novametrics managed the secretariat and led the data analysis, writing and production of this report with support from UNFPA, WHO, the Burnet Institute, ICM, the University of Southampton and Jamia Hamdard.

SoWMy 2021 builds on previous reports in this series (Box 1.1) and the *State of the World's Nursing 2020* report *(16)*. It is aligned with the SDGs and other high-level political commitments and recommendations, including those of the UN High-Level Commission on Health Employment and Economic Growth *(17)*. Figure 1.1 highlights key SRMNAH workforce and midwifery milestones from 2011 to 2020.

To minimize the data collection burden on countries, two main data reporting mechanisms were used: the WHO National Health Workforce Accounts (NHWA) platform *(18)* and the ICM Global Midwives Associations Map Survey *(19)*. The NHWA platform, established in October 2017 as the WHO official reporting system for health

Figure 1.1 Key global SRMNAH workforce and midwifery milestones, 2011–2020

Strengthening nursing and midwifery, resolution WHA64.7 (Sixty-fourth World Health Assembly): WHO is mandated to support Member States in developing plans and targets, implementing interdisciplinary health workforce teams and strengthening data collection.

SoWMy 2014:
A Universal Pathway.
A Woman's Right to Health

Comprehensive Midwifery Programme Guidance: developed by UNFPA in collaboration with partners to assist in scaling up and/ or strengthening midwifery programmes at the national level.

Conducting an SRMNAH workforce assessment (H4+): guidance to support countries to collect, understand, present and use SRMNAH workforce data for policy and planning.

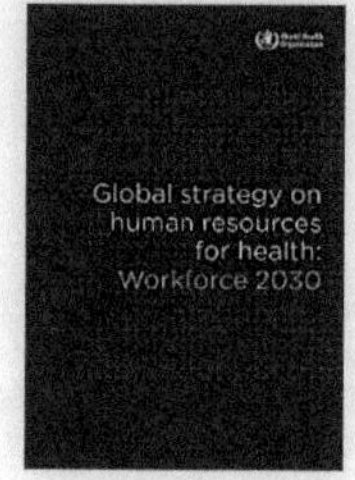

Global Strategy on Human Resources for Health: Workforce 2030 (WHO): primarily aimed at planners and policy-makers, this is relevant to all stakeholders in the health workforce.

2011 — 2014 — 2015 — 2016

SoWMy 2011: Delivering Health, Saving Lives

Strengthening midwifery toolkit (WHO): nine modules focus specifically on strengthening the central role and function of the professional midwife in providing high-quality SRMNAH care.

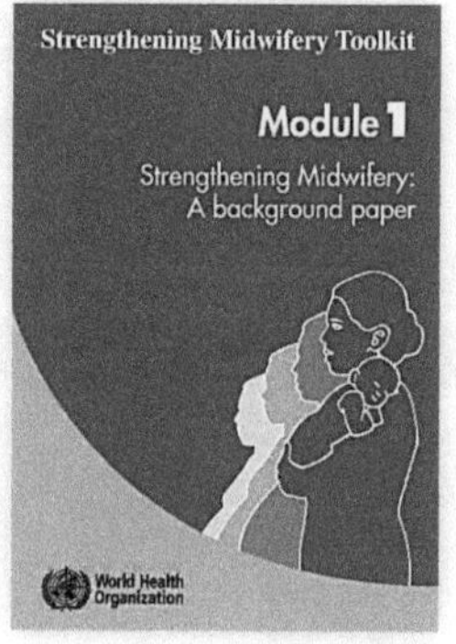

The Lancet Series on Midwifery: four papers update key aspects of midwifery, offering an evidence-based framework centring on the needs of women and their newborns and demonstrating the key role of midwives in reducing maternal and perinatal mortality.

Strengthening nursing and midwifery, resolution WHA67.24 (Sixty-seventh World Health Assembly): Member States renew commitments to UHC and request the Director-General to develop a new global strategy for human resources for health.

Global Strategy for Women's, Children's and Adolescents' Health (2016–2030): objectives are to achieve the highest attainable standard of health for all women, children and adolescents, transform the future and ensure that every newborn, mother and child not only survives, but thrives.

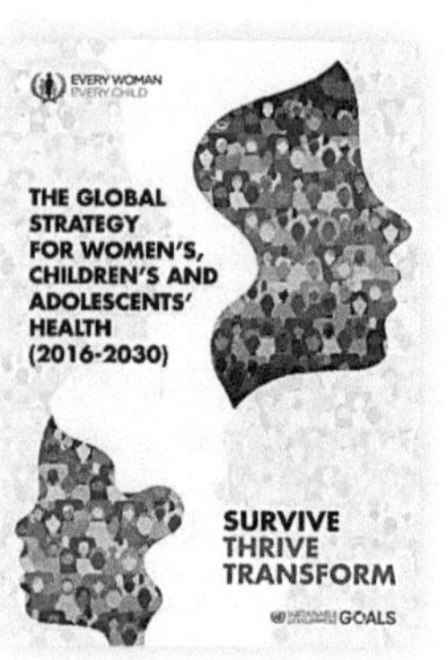

Global strategic directions for strengthening nursing and midwifery, 2016–2020 (WHO): identifies four areas of strategic focus: education and training, leadership and governance, interdisciplinary collaboration and political will for workforce development.

Midwives' Voices, Midwives' Realities (WHO): 2,470 midwives in 93 countries describe the barriers they experience in providing high-quality, respectful care for women, newborns and their families.

Marla E Kristian examines Meliana, in Makassar, Indonesia.
© Bill & Melinda Gates Foundation/Prashant Panjiar.

workforce statistics, is updated on an ongoing basis with government-validated data that have been checked for consistency. The ICM survey was completed by professional midwife associations (or, in countries with no such association, by the UNFPA country office) and validated by the competent national authorities. Other data sources included a WHO Policy Survey *(20)*. This is a different data collection process from that used in previous SoWMy reports, which restricts the extent to which we can analyse workforce trends over time. Full details of the data collection can be found in Webappendix 2.

All 194 WHO Member States were eligible for inclusion in SoWMy 2021, and all submitted at least one data item that is featured in this report. Each piece of analysis is based on a different number of countries, reflecting the differing levels of data availability for individual indicators. Each table and figure shows the number of reporting countries; Webappendix 4 shows which countries provided data for each piece of analysis.

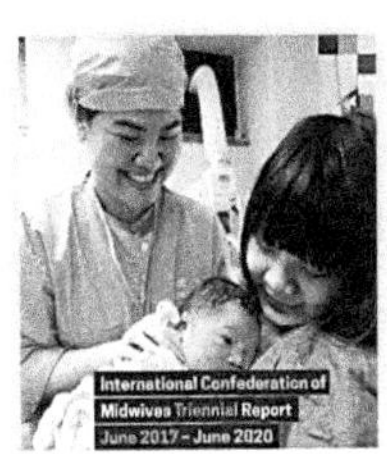

International Confederation of Midwives: ICM publishes its strategic directions for the triennium 2017–2020, focusing on quality, equity and leadership.

Global Midwifery Strategy 2018–2030 (UNFPA): developed to advance the attainment of SDG 3, the strategy aims to help reduce the global maternal mortality ratio to less than 70 deaths per 100,000 live births by 2030.

Strengthening quality midwifery education for universal health coverage 2030: framework for action: developed by WHO, UNFPA, UNICEF and ICM, the report includes a seven-step action plan for use by all stakeholders in maternal and newborn health.

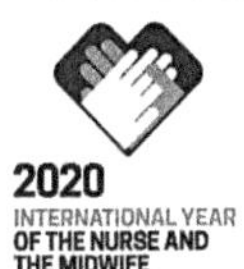

International Year of the Nurse and the Midwife (designated by the World Health Assembly).

State of the World's Nursing 2020: Investing in Education, Jobs and Leadership.

| 2017 | 2018 | 2019 | 2020 |

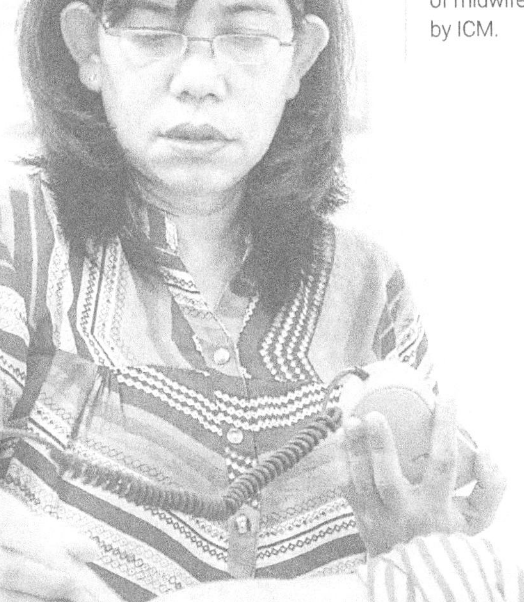

Essential competencies for midwifery practice 2018 update (ICM): outlines the minimum set of knowledge, skills and professional behaviours required to use the designation of midwife as defined by ICM.

Essential competencies for midwifery practice 2019 update (ICM): includes midwives' role in preventing, detecting and stabilizing complications.

8th WHO-ICM-ICN Triad Meeting: participants commit to support countries in developing and implementing 10 priority actions to advance nursing and midwifery agendas in response to the Covid-19 pandemic and towards the realization of UHC.

Seventy-third World Health Assembly: designated 2021 as the International Year of Health and Care Workers.

Impact of midwives paper in *The Lancet Global Health:* study led by ICM, UNFPA and WHO provides new estimates on midwives' potential to reduce maternal and neonatal mortality and stillbirths.

The first part of this report focuses specifically on midwives, given the unique and central role they play not only in maternity care but across the entire continuum of SRMNAH care. Chapter 2 shows why countries should invest more in midwives, and Chapter 3 presents data on progress and barriers/challenges relating to midwifery education, regulation and legislation. Chapter 4 assesses the need for and availability of midwives and other SRMNAH workers at global and regional levels and by income group, and Chapter 5 focuses on equity of access to the SRMNAH workforce. Chapter 6 considers how to enable and empower the SRMNAH workforce, highlighting a number of gender-related issues, including leadership and decent work. Finally, Chapter 7 assesses progress since SoWMy 2011 and sets out actions to ensure that midwives play a central role in the interdisciplinary teams needed to provide integrated, high-quality SRMNAH care.

SoWMy 2021's two-page country profiles (see https://unfpa.org/sowmy) provide detailed national-level data on the SRMNAH workforce and the environment in which it operates.

The devastating effects of Covid-19 on women, newborns and adolescents, as well as on the SRMNAH workforce, are highlighted throughout this report. Health professionals have shown huge commitment despite the increased risks to their own health due to numerous deficiencies in the management of the health workforce *(21)*. Governments and relevant stakeholders are urged to use SoWMy 2021 to inform their efforts to build back better and fairer from the pandemic, forging stronger primary health-care systems as a pathway to UHC and fostering a more equitable world for all *(22)*. It is hoped that the pandemic will be a catalyst for change given the heightened profile of health workers. SoWMy 2021 can help make this happen.

Midwives, nurses, doctors and students at a staff meeting in Labasa Hospital, Fiji.
© Felicity Copeland.

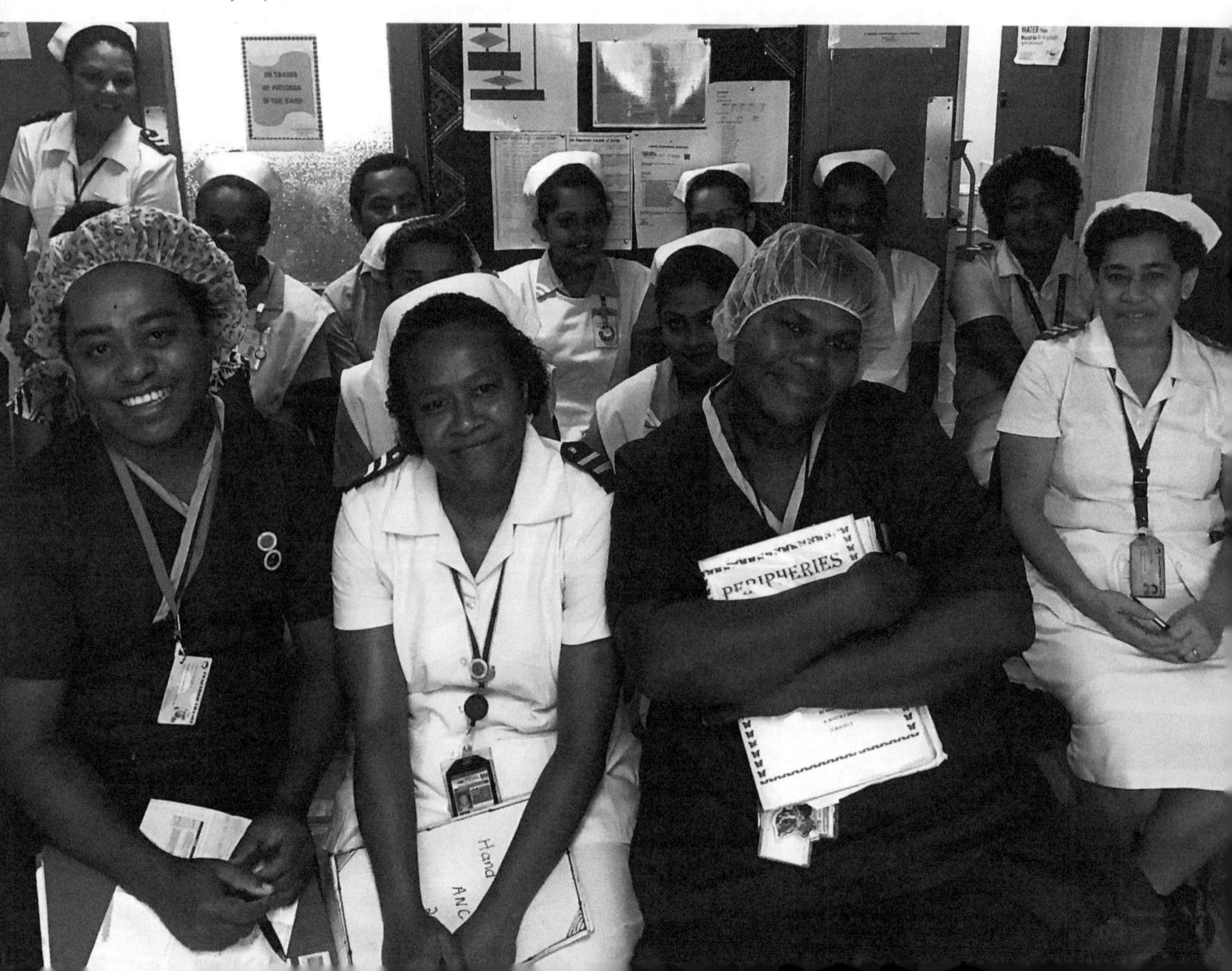

MIDWIVES: A VITAL INVESTMENT

CHAPTER 2

Midwives provide many essential clinical SRMNAH interventions and can play a broader role in activities such as advancing primary health care and UHC, responding to violence against women, and addressing sexual and reproductive rights *(29)*. They can be a point-of-contact in the community for sexual and reproductive health services, including contraception, comprehensive abortion care, and screening for and treatment of sexually transmitted infections, human papillomavirus and intimate partner violence. Midwives play a vital role in resuscitating newborns, promoting breastfeeding and supporting the mother and the family in infant care. Midwives also support and promote self-care interventions, for example, self-management of nutritional supplements and self-monitoring of blood glucose and blood pressure during pre-pregnancy and the antenatal and postnatal periods, and can support self-managed medical abortion. Midwives can support implementation of rights-based and gender-transformative approaches for women living with HIV, and advocate to prevent female genital mutilation and other harmful practices.

In addition to their clinical roles, midwives also work in education institutions, management, policy, research, regulation, midwives' associations and government. It is important to count and value midwives working in these areas, which are fundamentally important for the development of the profession. Strengthening midwifery at a country level requires multilevel investments, including in those who educate and support midwives in clinical practice and ensure the delivery of high-quality care.

Impact of midwives

Analysis conducted as part of SoWMy 2021 showed that midwives can help substantially reduce maternal and neonatal mortality and stillbirths in low- and middle-income countries. This analysis of the 88 countries that account for the vast majority of the world's maternal and neonatal deaths and stillbirths showed that a substantial increase in coverage of midwife-delivered interventions (25% increase every five years to 2035) could avert 40% of maternal and newborn deaths and 26% of stillbirths *(30)*. Even a modest increase (10% every five years) in coverage of midwife-delivered interventions could avert 23% of maternal and neonatal deaths and 14% of stillbirths. Universal coverage of

---

KEY MESSAGES

▶ Midwives, when educated, licensed and fully integrated in and supported by interdisciplinary teams, and in an enabling environment, can provide a wide range of clinical interventions and contribute to broader health goals, such as advancing primary health care, addressing sexual and reproductive rights, promoting self-care interventions and empowering women.

▶ Midwives play a vital role in preventing maternal and newborn deaths and stillbirths: increasing access to competent and regulated midwives could save millions of lives each year.

▶ The wide range of contributions that midwives can make to SRMNAH and broader health goals makes them an obvious focus for investment.

▶ The evidence indicates that investing in midwives facilitates positive birth experiences, improves health outcomes, augments workforce supply, favours inclusive and equitable growth, facilitates economic stabilization, and can have a positive macroeconomic impact.

midwife-delivered interventions would avert 65% of maternal and neonatal deaths and stillbirths.

Midwife-led care that includes continuity of care produces additional benefits (see glossary and Box 2.1). A systematic review of 15 studies involving 17,674 mothers and newborns from four high-income countries showed benefits in terms of outcomes, satisfaction and potential cost savings *(31)*. Another systematic review showed that organizational reforms in maternity services that promote midwife-led continuity of care reduce caesarean section rates *(32)*.

Previous research through *The Lancet* Series on Midwifery showed more than 50 short-, medium- and long-term outcomes that could be improved by care within a midwife's scope of practice. These include: reduced maternal and neonatal mortality and morbidity, fewer stillbirths and preterm births, fewer unnecessary interventions, and improved psychosocial and public health outcomes such as reduced anxiety and increased uptake of contraception and immunization *(33)*.

The way in which women and newborns receive care during childbirth makes a difference to their health outcomes. The structure and organization of health-care systems and the economic, social and cultural contexts in which they operate differ widely between countries, in turn influencing the models of maternity care available to women. The ICM Midwifery Services Framework *(34)* can be used to support workforce development.

Some low- and middle-income countries that are already on the path to achieving targeted reductions in their maternal mortality ratio (MMR) have significantly increased midwives' role as key attendants for normal births over the last two decades *(42)*.

Despite resource constraints, 28 low- and lower-middle-income countries reduced their MMR by more than 50% between 2000 and 2017 *(2)*. Figure 2.1 examines recent changes in 18 of these countries that have data: many have increased deployment of midwives or nurses at births, usually in facilities. For instance, Malawi's MMR fell by more than 50% between 2000 and 2017 (down from

Midwife-led continuity of care

Midwife-led continuity of care (MLCC) models, in which a known midwife or small group of known midwives supports a woman throughout the antenatal, intrapartum and postnatal continuum, are recommended for pregnant women in settings with well functioning midwifery programmes *(35)*. In high-income countries, MLCC models have been shown to lead to reductions in neonatal deaths, preterm births *(36)*, epidural, episiotomy or instrumental births, and to increases in spontaneous vaginal birth and women's satisfaction, with no increased risk of harm *(31)*. Investment in midwives to achieve these outcomes is cost-effective *(37, 38)*. MLCC enables each woman and her midwife (or small team of midwives) to get to know each other and to build a relationship based on trust, equity, informed choice, shared decision-making and shared responsibility *(39, 40)*. Relationships are negotiated between the partners, and are dynamic and empowering for both *(41)*.

Current evidence for MLCC comes mainly from high-income countries. Implementing and scaling up MLCC models sustainably requires addressing the challenges to midwives' education, regulation and working environments described in this report. This can lead to improved health outcomes, not only for women and newborns, but also for their families and societies.

Contributed by Sally Pairman (ICM).

749 to 349 deaths per 100,000 live births) while the percentage of births in a health facility increased by 83% and the percentage of midwife/nurse-assisted births increased by 36%. The Association of Malawian Midwives cited the national maternal and newborn health road map *(43)* as a significant contribution to this achievement.[2] Box 2.2 describes how Cambodia (a lower-middle-income country) achieved positive results, and also features the Netherlands, a high-income country with a strong midwifery profession that continues to drive down its MMR.

Multiple returns from investing in midwives

A strong health system is essential for achieving UHC and ensuring progress towards the SDGs. While the health workforce is a core element of the health system, it often turns out to be its weakest link as it is usually perceived as driving costs, rather than producing positive health and social outcomes. Maximizing midwives' impact, improving the quality of SRMNAH care and addressing the workforce shortages reported in Chapter 4 will require significant financial outlay. However, there is growing recognition that creating jobs for health workers not only bolsters population health but also supports sustainable economic growth and progress towards other SDGs.

Discussion of the economic and broader social benefits of investments in health has in recent years focused on the concept of "the investment case", arguing in favour of investment. The key term "investment" reflects the fact that the benefits of an adequate health workforce outweigh the costs of their education, training and employment.

FIGURE 2.1 **Change in % of births in facilities and % of births attended by midwives and nurses in 18 low-income and lower-middle-income countries that reduced their maternal mortality ratio by more than 50% between 2000 and 2017**

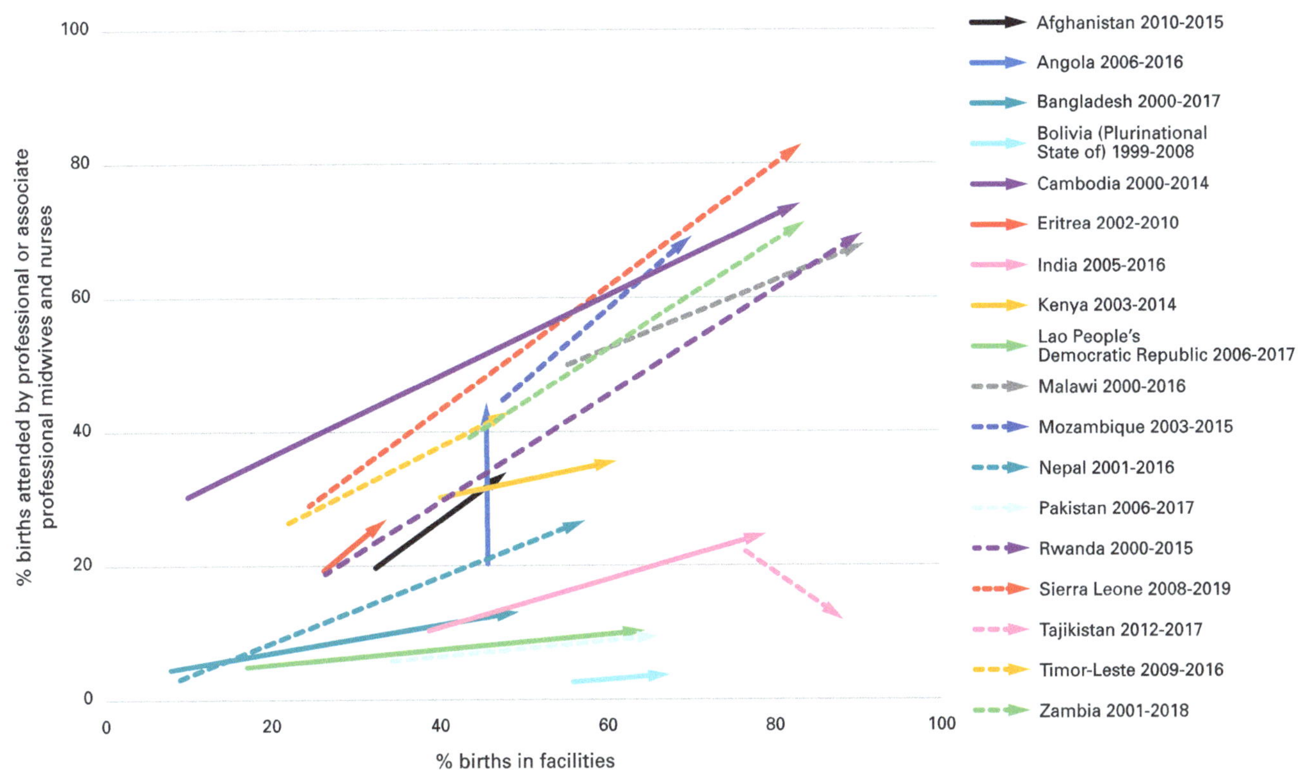

Source: DHS STATcompiler (44) and individual DHS reports.

2 Phoya A, Association of Malawian Midwives, Personal communication, 2020.

Investment in midwives in Cambodia and the Netherlands

Cambodia

Nearly 1,500 public health facilities in Cambodia offer comprehensive SRMNAH services, with at least one midwife at each facility. Outreach activities are carried out in hard-to-reach locations, with essential medicines, equipment and materials being provided to health facilities. Cambodia's MMR dropped from 488 deaths per 100,000 live births in 2000 to 160 in 2017; the figure below illustrates the policies that have been implemented since 2000.

Births in Cambodia, by type of birth attendant, 2000–2014

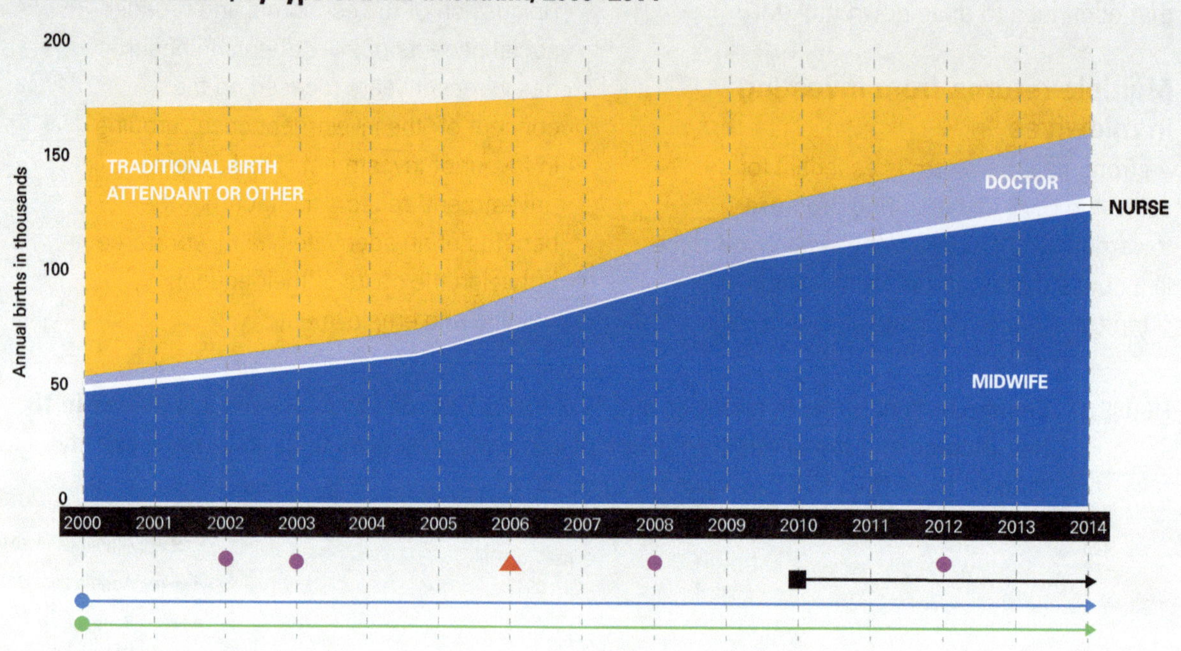

Source: DHS reports from 2000, 2005, 2010 and 2014 and World Population Prospects 2019.

EXPAND ACCESS

From the late 1990s onwards Cambodia introduced mechanisms including vouchers and equity fund exemptions. The "Health Equity Fund" was set up in 2019 to provide over 2.4 million poor people with free access to services across the country. Additional cash support is given to poor pregnant women for maternal and newborn health care from pregnancy to 1,000 days after birth.

QUALITY OF CARE

Competency-based midwifery curricula have been further developed with clinical labs, clinical practice and adult-based learning approaches, including simulation and scenario-based learning for students. The Government Midwifery Incentive Scheme drove a dramatic increase in numbers of births and quality of care at health facilities in the 2000s, contributing to decreases in maternal death rates *(45)*.

EDUCATION

In 2002, a post-basic midwifery programme was introduced (3 years' nursing plus 1 year midwifery). In 2003, the Ministry of Health introduced a 1-year interim Primary Nurse-Midwife course, designed to address severe shortages of midwives. In 2008, a 3-year direct-entry Associate Degree in Midwifery was introduced, and in 2012, a 4-year direct-entry BSc in Midwifery started to be offered at public and private schools. A bridging curriculum from Associate Degree to BSc has produced 50 graduates.

REGULATION

In 2006, the Cambodia Midwives Council was established, in addition to the Cambodian Midwives Association which was established in 1994. In 2016, licensing and relicensing were introduced to protect the title "midwife".

DEPLOYMENT

Midwives deployed at midwifery-led care units increased from 3,678 in 2010 to 7,128 in 2019 (in addition to the 6,463 midwives educated under the old curricula).

Contributed by Chea Ath (Cambodia Midwives Association) and Sokun Sok, Sopha Muong and Pros Nguon (UNFPA Cambodia).

The Netherlands

Midwives in the Netherlands work independently in the community in group practices, or in hospitals. Women refer themselves to a midwife for maternity care. Community midwives provide care in several ways: at health facility outpatient centres, in a birthing centre, in hospital, or at home (transferring to obstetrician-led care when necessary). Both community and hospital midwives assist women during normal births in facilities. Births with a midwife now account for over 75% of all women giving birth, and midwives are the sole caregiver in 57% *(46)*. Despite a decreasing birth rate, the option to receive care by a midwife regardless of the setting has kept midwifery at the centre of health system development for maternal and newborn health *(46)*. The country's MMR dropped from 13 per 100,000 live births in 2000 to 5 in 2017.

Births attended by midwives in the Netherlands, by birth setting, 2010–2019

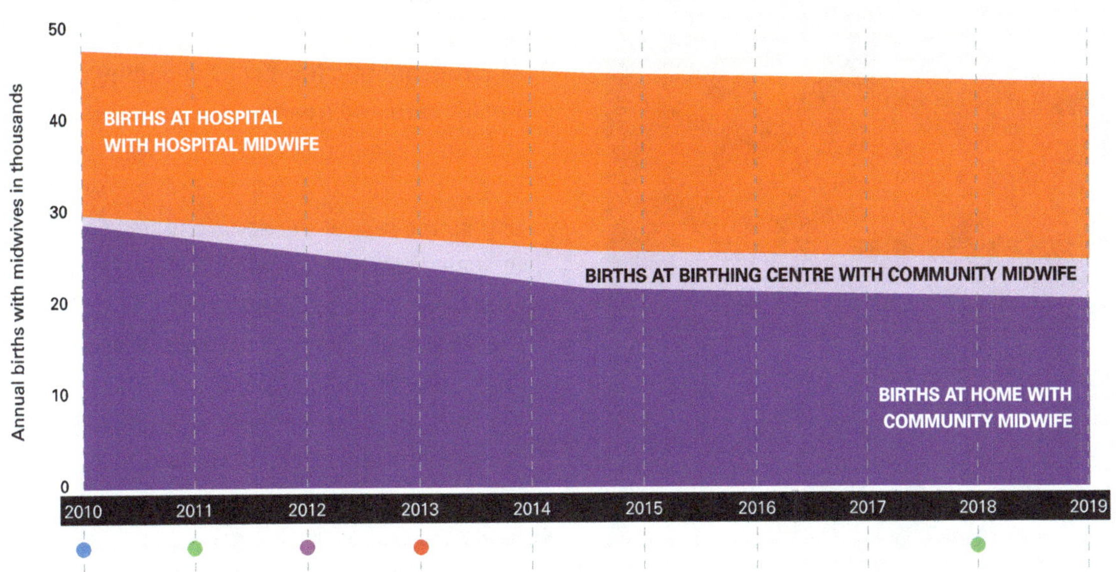

Source: Ank de Jonge, Marianne Nieuwenhuijze, Bob Radder.

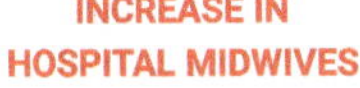

EDUCATION

Midwifery education is a direct-entry, 4-year BSc programme, which includes the midwife's public health role, interprofessional collaboration, shared decision-making and expanded scope of practice, helping to position midwives as a strong, autonomous partner in care for women and newborns. An MSc was created in 2001 to bridge the gap between BSc and research opportunities for midwives, and in 2010 institutions created PhD programmes.

WOMEN'S ACCESS TO CARE BY A MIDWIFE

To address differences in access to care, "Healthy Pregnancy 4 All" and "Promising Start" were initiated in 2011 *(47)* and 2018 *(48)*, providing support for specific challenges (e.g. debt, lack of social network, unsafe situations) that may confront women in vulnerable circumstances, including migrant women.

QUALITY OF CARE

In 2006, the national midwives' organization (KNOV) developed a voluntary quality register that most midwives joined in addition to the existing government register which protects the title "midwife". According to KNOV's monitoring system, group antenatal care was implemented in three midwifery practices. By 2012, 143 midwifery practices offered this approach, with the aim of reducing over-medicalization.

INCREASE IN HOSPITAL MIDWIVES

In 2008, 75% of the 1,763 registered midwives worked as independent practitioners in community settings and 25% as hospital midwives *(49)*. By 2012, an estimated 77% of hospital births under the responsibility of an obstetrician were attended by hospital midwives and 40% were solely managed by a midwife. By 2013, there were 23 home-like birth centres accessible to low-risk women supported by a community midwife. Of these centres, three were free-standing, 14 operated alongside an obstetric unit and six were integrated in an obstetric unit.

Contributed by Ank de Jonge, Marianne Nieuwenhuijze and Bob Radder (KNOV).

Despite evidence that the health system and the health workforce are areas in which social investment is effective, the number of studies assessing the benefits (sometimes called the return on investment) for the health workforce generally, and specifically for midwives, remains limited. To better understand the different kinds of benefits produced by such investments, WHO has reviewed, analysed and synthesized evidence on this issue. This work identified five key resulting benefits:

1. **Health outcomes.** There is strong evidence that investing in midwives leads to better health outcomes by reducing maternal and neonatal deaths and stillbirths *(30)*.

2. **Improved labour supply and level of economic activity.** An improved supply of midwives contributes to increased economic activity.

3. **Macroeconomic impact of spending on health care and health-care workers.** Investment in health care and health-care workers produces significant multipliers across the rest of the economy. Studies indicate that these multipliers can be greater than those produced by investment in other economic sectors, making investment in health care and health-care workers particularly attractive, especially for public-sector decision-makers.

4. **Inclusive and equitable growth.** Investing in midwives provides an opportunity to increase women's employment and the availability of decent work.

5. **Economic stabilization.** Various studies note that, in an economic downturn, the number of people employed in health care tends to decline less than in other sectors. Such continued spending acts as an economic stabilizer in difficult times and also serves to maintain standards of care.

There is no "one size fits all" approach to assessing the benefits and returns on investment in health-care workers, including midwives. Different approaches are possible, each with its own strengths and limitations.

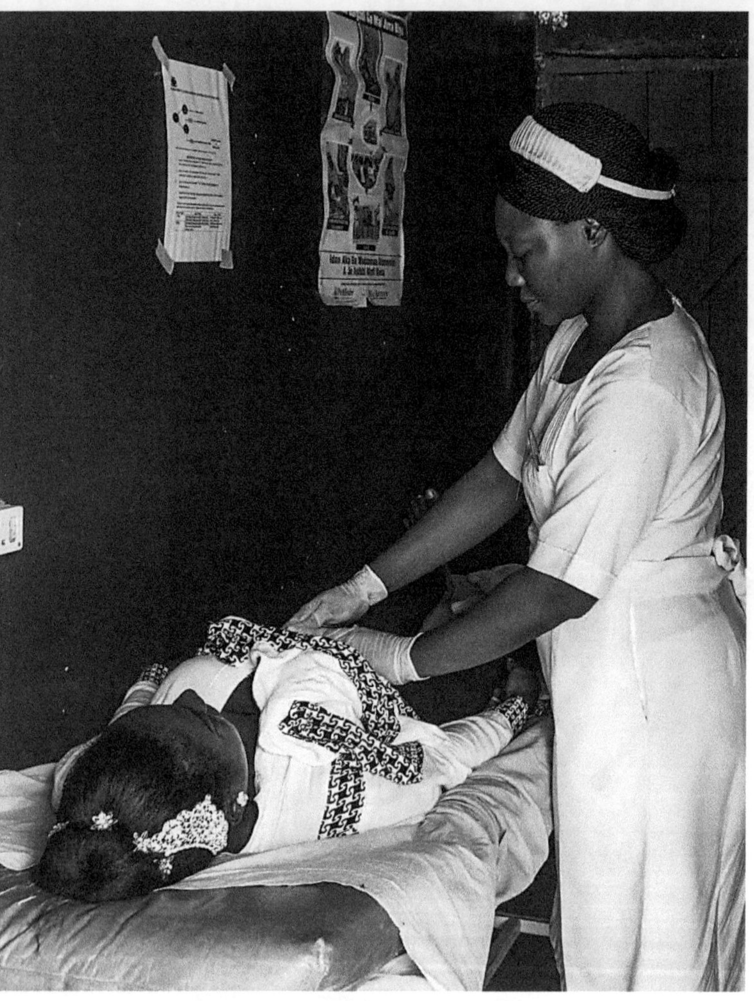

A midwife performs an antenatal check for Mercy Yakubu at the Primary Health Care Centre in Akwanga, Nasarawa State, Nigeria. © Gates Archive/Nelson Owoicho.

EDUCATION AND REGULATION OF MIDWIVES TO ENSURE HIGH-QUALITY CARE

CHAPTER 3

Education

High-quality midwifery education is essential to prepare midwives to provide high-quality SRMNAH care *(50)*. Despite evidence of the benefits produced by investment in it, midwifery education and training remain grossly under-funded in many countries. There are wide variations in the content, quality and duration of education programmes, and key challenges relating to resources and infrastructure which adversely affect students' learning experience and limit opportunities for gaining "hands-on" experience *(51-56)*. Research across Africa and South Asia has shown that inadequate education and training significantly jeopardize the professional identity, competence and confidence of midwives as primary SRMNAH care providers *(57)*. However, there are indications that positive efforts to improve the quality of midwifery education are under way in a number of countries *(58)*, including India (Box 3.1).

In 2019, UNFPA, UNICEF, WHO and ICM identified three strategic priorities for midwifery education: every woman and newborn to be cared for by a midwife, educated and trained to international standards and enabled to legally practice the full scope of midwifery, and the title "midwife" to be used only for providers who are educated to international standards; midwifery leadership to be positioned in high-level national policy, planning and budgeting processes to improve decision-making about investments for midwifery education to help achieve UHC; and coordination and alignment between midwifery stakeholders at global, regional and country levels to align education and training processes, knowledge, research, evidence-based materials, indicators and investment *(51)*.

The ICM member association survey described in Chapter 1 and Webappendix 2 collected data from 80 countries on their midwife education programmes: 33 (41%) offer only direct-entry programmes, 17 (21%) offer only post-nursing, five (6%) offer combined nursing and midwifery and 25 (31%) offer both direct-entry and another type of programme.

🔑 KEY MESSAGES

- ▸ **The quality of pre-service midwifery education needs to be improved. Key challenges include the lack of investment in educators, limited skills and knowledge in contemporary teaching and learning, inadequate "hands-on" experience for students and gaps in infrastructure, resources and systems, particularly in low- and middle-income countries.**

- ▸ **Covid-19 has prompted new ways of providing midwifery education and services. These need to be developed and used effectively, including innovative digital technologies and online learning opportunities. Their effectiveness also needs to be assessed during "normal" conditions.**

- ▸ **Nearly all (91%) of 74 responding countries reported that they offered midwifery qualification to bachelor's degree level or higher. However, on average only two-thirds of midwife educators are themselves qualified midwives, and there are challenges to the provision of high-quality education.**

- ▸ **In many countries, midwives are not authorized to perform tasks typically considered part of the midwife's scope of practice. This is most common in the Americas, European and the Eastern Mediterranean regions, and in high-income countries.**

Of the 63 countries reporting a direct-entry midwifery programme or a combined midwifery and nursing programme, 53 have a programme of at least three years' duration, of which 23 last longer than three years. Figure 3.1 shows that programmes of at least three years' duration are the norm in all WHO regions *(60)* and World Bank income groups *(61)*, but the small number of reporting countries in some regions and income groups means that these results are not necessarily representative of all countries in that region or group. Programmes lasting four to five years are most common in South-East Asia and in upper-middle-income countries. Of the 41 countries reporting a post-nursing midwifery education pathway, 30 report that it is at least 18 months in duration, but eight countries report a one-year programme and three countries have a programme lasting less than one year.

Of 175 responding countries in NHWA, 79% reported a master list of accredited health worker education institutions, and a further 7% have a partial list, leaving 14% without such a list. ICM has developed a Midwifery Education Accreditation Programme *(62)* to support the development of accreditation processes (Box 3.2).

There is also variation in education standards. Of 57 responding countries in NHWA (of which just two were low-income countries), 93% had standards for the duration and content of midwifery professional education and 86%

The Government of India's Midwifery Initiative

Under the Midwifery Initiative, with its vision to provide midwife-led care services in public health facilities, the Government of India launched *Guidelines on Midwifery Services* in December 2018. Its aim is to create a cohort of Nurse Practitioners in Midwifery, capable of providing positive birth experiences to women by promoting physiological birth (thus reducing over-medicalization), providing respectful maternity care, and decongesting higher-level health facilities by providing services in midwife-led care units. The focus is on ensuring empowerment and improved career progression for midwives.

India has identified seven National Training Institutes of Excellence for training midwifery educators. In 2019, the Ministry of Health and Family Welfare initiated midwifery educator training at one of these Institutes. Post-training, midwifery services will initially be provided in tertiary and secondary health facilities; in subsequent phases it will be made available in primary health centres as part of a comprehensive primary health-care package.

To support the implementation of the Midwifery Initiative, the Government, with WHO, commissioned a study in six states to assess the midwifery competencies of practitioners and educators, and research on barriers to and facilitators for high-quality midwifery services. Survey tools were based on the ICM essential competencies for midwifery practice and the WHO midwifery educator core competencies. Barriers were examined with a focus on India and South-East Asia, as well as at the global level. The study identified barriers and facilitators relating to: education, training, supervision, deployment, lack of recognition of midwifery as an autonomous profession, and lack of appropriate roles enabling midwives to work to their full scope of practice. In terms of service provision, barriers included low coverage and quality of some services, poor working environments, and lack of equipment and supplies. The main recommendation was to implement a high-quality pre-service education programme to prepare midwives who are competent, meet global standards and are able to provide high-quality, evidence-based care *(59)*.

Based on the research and information collected, the Government, in collaboration with stakeholders including the Indian Nursing Council, developed a strategic roadmap for effective rollout of the Midwifery Initiative. The roadmap includes a curriculum, scope and standards of practice, advocacy toolkits and learning resource packages for both the Midwifery Educator programme and the Nurse Practitioners in Midwifery programme, with the objective of raising midwifery education and service provision to global standards.

Contributed by Ministry of Health and Family Welfare, Government of India.

Duration of direct-entry midwifery or combined nursing and midwifery education programmes in 63 countries, by WHO region and World Bank income group, 2019–2020

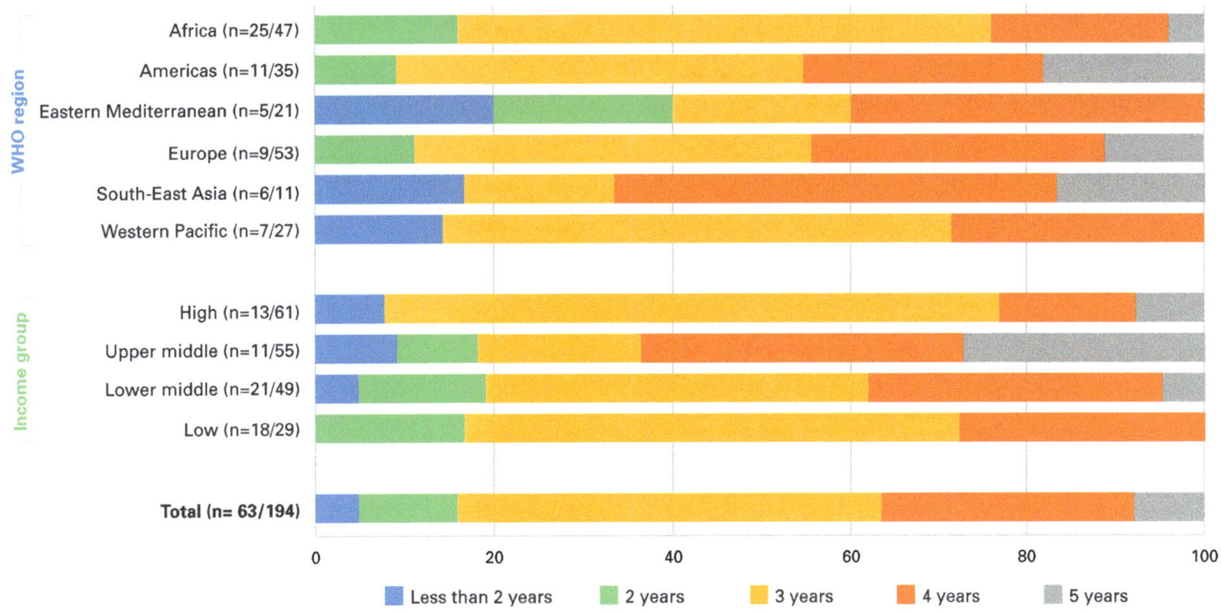

Note: Many countries reported more than one type of direct-entry or combined education programme: in those cases, only the longest programme is included in this graph.

Source: ICM survey.

The ICM Midwifery Education Accreditation Programme

The ICM Midwifery Education Accreditation Programme (MEAP) is based on international best practices in midwifery education and accreditation. It evaluates pre-service midwifery educational programmes against the ICM *Global Standards for Midwifery Education* (2013 and subsequent updates), including competency-based education that in turn includes ICM's *Essential Competencies for Midwifery Practice* (updated in 2019).

The MEAP serves as a benchmark for midwifery educational programmes that aim to meet international standards. For a fee, it offers accreditation approval based on an independent assessment of an institute's midwifery educational programme(s) to determine the extent to which ICM standards are met *(63)*. It also helps to identify best practices and gaps, allowing donors and implementers to provide targeted, effective and

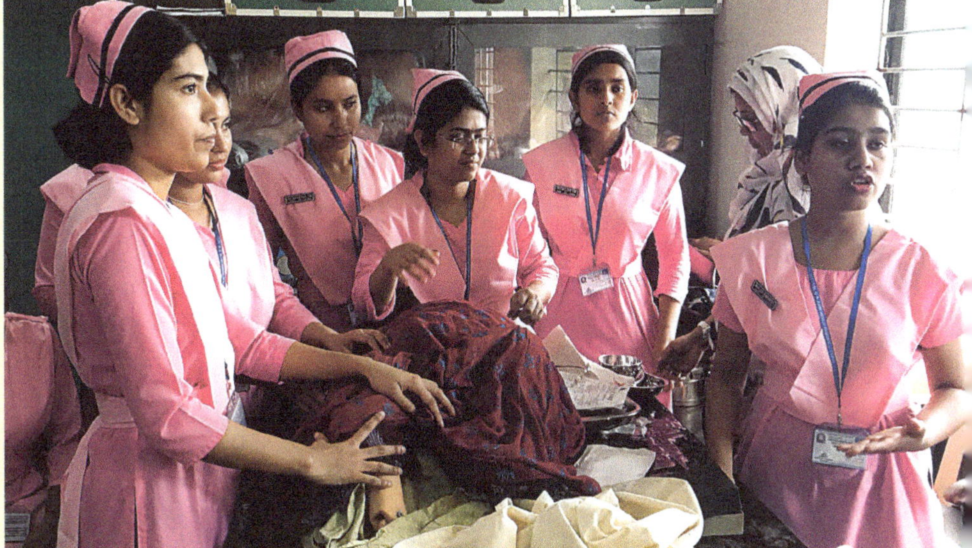
Midwifery students in Mymensingh, Bangladesh. © UNFPA/Geeta Lal.

sustainable support for high-quality midwifery education.

ICM commenced assessing midwifery programmes using MEAP in 2020. Its first accreditation was of a direct-entry midwifery programme in Rwanda. In response to travel restrictions due to the Covid-19 pandemic, ICM is adapting MEAP for implementation using digital technologies and other solutions.

Contributed by Sally Pairman (ICM).

had accreditation mechanisms for midwifery professional education institutions.

Of 70 reporting countries, 34 (49%) reported that **all** their midwife educators are qualified midwives, and four (6%) reported that **none** of their midwife educators are midwives. On **average** in the 70 reporting countries, 65% of midwife educators were midwives. Figure 3.2 shows that this percentage is highest in the European, Eastern Mediterranean and South-East Asia regions, and lowest in Africa. Again, however, small numbers of reporting countries may mean these results are not fully representative of the regions. High-income countries are more likely than middle- and low-income countries to use midwives to teach midwifery. This may result from lack of support and pathways for midwives to become educators *(64, 65)*. Box 3.3 describes the findings of a WHO survey of midwifery educators, which highlighted some of the specific challenges they face in low- and middle-income countries.

Of 74 reporting countries, over one third (38%) reported that the highest level of midwifery qualification available was a bachelor's degree, one quarter (26%) said a master's-level qualification was the highest available, and another quarter (27%) offered a doctorate-level programme. For just under one in 10 countries (9%) the highest level was below degree level. Figure 3.3 shows that master's- and doctorate-level midwifery qualifications are most likely to be available in Europe and in high-income countries, but again the small number of reporting countries in some regions means that these results should be interpreted with caution.

Regulation and association

Each country's midwifery regulation governs the education, practice and licensure of its midwives. National laws and regulations establish who is qualified to use the title "midwife", as well as the midwife's scope of practice. Midwives' associations are established at country level to support

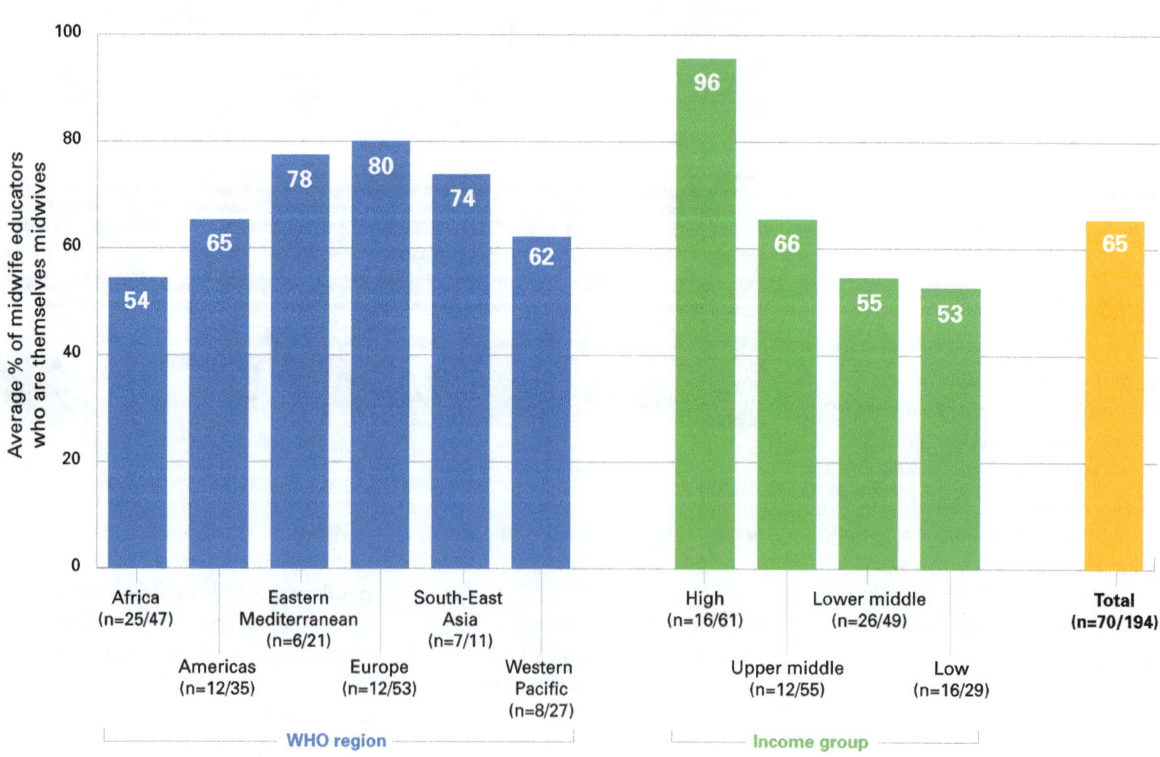

Figure 3.2 **Average % of midwife educators who are themselves midwives in 70 countries, by WHO region and World Bank income group, 2019–2020**

Source: ICM survey.

Key data on quality of education from WHO's global midwifery educator survey

In 2018–2019, WHO conducted a global midwifery educator survey, collecting the views of those actively teaching midwifery (midwives, nurses, doctors) in low- and middle-income countries across five of the six WHO regions (excepting Europe). The purpose was to better understand the actions needed to improve the quality of midwifery education. Over 100 educational institutions in 35 countries responded. Key challenges identified included the following:

- Across all educational institutions, respondents indicated that regulation of education programmes did not effectively ensure quality nor facilitate standardization in midwifery education; varying levels of skills were being taught through differing pathways.
- Just over half of the respondents indicated that their profession was midwifery. Fewer than half were trained or accredited as educators.

- Just over half of institutions had knowledge of and access to WHO Midwifery Education Modules and other education materials.
- Educators had greatest confidence in their ability to teach care of the woman and baby during labour and childbirth, followed by antenatal care and emergency obstetric care. They had least confidence in their ability to teach family planning and newborn care, especially care of small and sick newborns. None of the respondents felt confident in all of WHO's midwifery educator core competencies.
- 100% of educators reported shortages of at least some equipment and supplies in classrooms, skills labs and/or clinical settings.
- All educators, except those in the Americas region, experienced challenges relating to water, sanitation and hygiene. The challenges are greatest in Africa

(especially in French-speaking countries) where three quarters of educators said they lacked access to clean water at least some of the time. Many educators in Africa and South-East Asia reported not having access to a functioning toilet in their workplace.

This survey gives an indication of the nature and scale of the challenges faced by many midwife educators and provides a basis to guide research and action. The survey findings were a vital input to the joint WHO, UNFPA, UNICEF and ICM "Framework for action for strengthening quality midwifery education for UHC 2030" *(51)* which aims to ensure that the education system produces midwives who are confident and competent to fulfil their potential to ensure that mothers and newborns survive and thrive.

Contributed by Fran McConville (WHO).

Figure 3.3 **Highest level of midwifery qualification available in 74 countries, by WHO region and World Bank income group, 2019–2020**

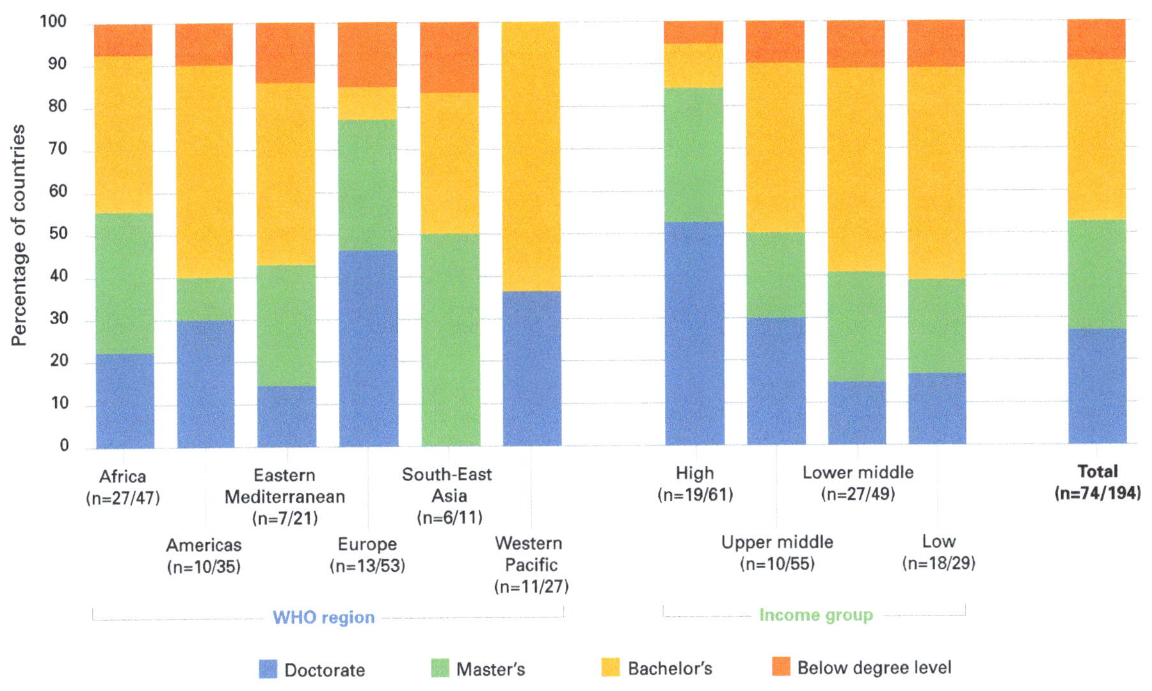

Source: ICM survey.

members of the profession and to provide leadership to strengthen and advance the role and impact of midwives. They should be separate from the regulators of midwifery. Some associations also function as a trade union.

Of the countries providing data, three quarters (77%) indicated that their country had legislation recognizing midwifery as distinct from nursing, including over 90% of responding countries in the Americas, European and Western Pacific regions (Table 3.1).

Table 3.1 also shows that three quarters (77%) of responding countries have at least one professional association specifically for midwives, and that this is the norm in all regions except South-East Asia.

Of 78 reporting countries, nearly all (92%) have a regulation system that covers midwives. One in eight (12%) reported a separate regulatory body specific to midwives. Most reporting countries (62%) do not have a separate regulator, but do have regulatory authority with policies and processes specifically for midwives (Figure 3.4). In 19% of countries, midwives are regulated by a regulatory body that is not specific to midwifery and does not have distinct policies and processes for midwives.

Countries use a variety of terms to describe the legal right to practise as a midwife. Half (49%) of 79 responding countries have both a licensing system and a registration system that are separate and mandatory processes, a quarter (25%) have registration only, 13% have licensing

TABLE 3.1

Percentage of countries with legislation recognizing midwifery as distinct from nursing and with an association specifically for midwives, by WHO region and World Bank income group, 2019–2020

	Number of countries reporting/total	% of countries with legislation recognizing midwifery as distinct from nursing	Number of countries reporting/total	% of countries with an association specifically for midwives*
WHO REGION				
Africa	29/47	62%	35/47	77%
Americas	12/35	92%	17/35	88%
Eastern Mediterranean	7/21	86%	13/21	69%
Europe	13/53	92%	28/53	79%
South-East Asia	7/11	57%	8/11	50%
Western Pacific	11/27	91%	14/27	79%
INCOME GROUP				
High	19/61	89%	33/61	79%
Upper middle	12/55	92%	22/55	82%
Lower middle	28/49	68%	34/49	68%
Low	20/29	70%	26/29	81%
TOTAL	**79/194**	**77%**	**115**/194	**77%**

* The name of the association includes the word "midwife" (or equivalent term in the national language) and mentions no other health occupations. ** For this indicator only, the response of the midwives' association was accepted even without a validation letter, because the association was judged to be the competent authority to answer this question.

Source: ICM survey.

 Midwife regulation system in 78 countries, by WHO region and World Bank income group, 2019–2020

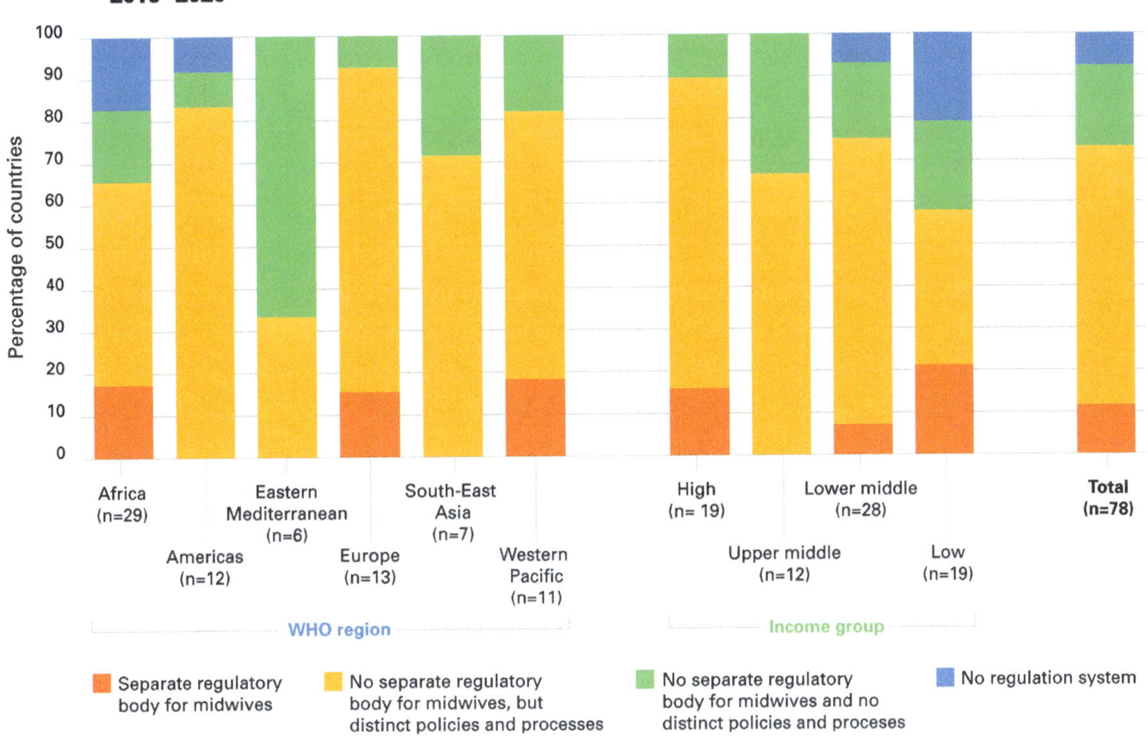

Source: ICM survey.

Figure 3.5 **Midwife licensing system in 73 countries, by WHO region and World Bank income group, 2019–2020**

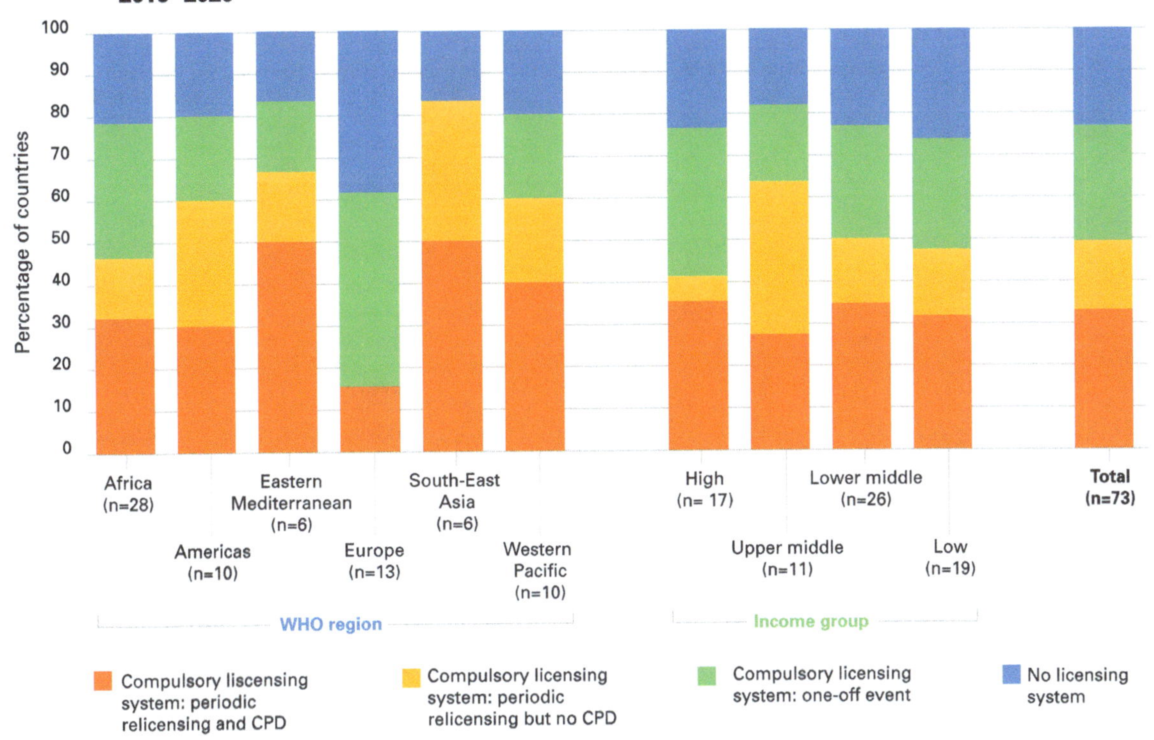

CPD = continuing professional development.

Source: ICM survey.

only and 12% have another type of system. Of 73 reporting countries, 17 have no licensing system at all, and 20 require their midwives to be licensed only once after qualifying, with no requirement for periodic renewal of the licence. The remaining 36 countries have a system involving periodic renewal, but only 24 of them require continuing professional development (Figure 3.5).

Licensing and regulatory systems are essential for safe practice, but not sufficient to maximize midwives' contribution to improved health outcomes. In many countries, midwives do not have the authority to perform tasks typically considered part of the midwife's scope of practice. For example, Table 3.2 shows that in most responding countries, midwives are authorized to provide five of the seven basic emergency obstetric and newborn care (BEmONC) signal functions, but in half of countries they are not authorized to undertake an instrumental birth using vacuum extraction or manual vacuum aspiration for early pregnancy bleeding.

Similarly, although WHO recommends that midwives can safely and effectively provide a wide range of contraceptive products *(66)*, some countries' regulatory systems restrict the range of products which midwives are authorized to provide. Table 3.3 shows that although most reporting countries authorize midwives to provide a wide range of contraceptive products, in some countries (mostly in the European and the Eastern Mediterranean regions) midwives are not authorized to provide such services.

Percentage of 79 countries in which midwives are authorized to provide BEmONC signal functions, by WHO region and World Bank income group, 2019–2020

	Number of countries reporting	Newborn resuscitation with bag and mask (%)	Oxytocics (%)	Parenteral antibiotics (%)	Anti-convulsants (%)	Manual removal of placenta (%)	Instrumental birth by vacuum extraction (%)	Manual vacuum aspiration %
WHO REGION								
Africa	29/47	100%	100%	100%	100%	97%	79%	90%
Americas	12/35	92%	100%	100%	83%	83%	17%	25%
Eastern Mediterranean	7/21	86%	57%	71%	57%	43%	57%	29%
Europe	13/53	100%	100%	85%	85%	46%	15%	8%
South-East Asia	7/11	100%	100%	86%	86%	71%	43%	57%
Western Pacific	11/27	100%	91%	91%	91%	71%	64%	36%
INCOME GROUP								
High	19/61	100%	100%	89%	79%	58%	26%	11%
Upper middle	12/55	83%	92%	92%	83%	58%	25%	25%
Lower middle	28/49	100%	96%	93%	93%	93%	64%	68%
Low	20/29	100%	90%	95%	95%	90%	75%	80%
TOTAL	**79/194**	**97%**	**95%**	**92%**	**89%**	**78%**	**52%**	**51%**

BEmONC = basic emergency obstetric and newborn care.

Source: ICM survey.

Impact of Covid-19 on midwives' education and practice

Covid-19 impacted on many activities in 2020 and 2021, including midwifery education and practice. Public health polices, including lockdowns, caused significant disruption to essential health services *(67)*. Midwifery education, like that of other health occupations, was also disrupted, with teaching moving online, limited access to clinical placements and changes in students' direct patient care contact hours *(68-71)*. In some settings, programmes and providers developed new digital solutions, increased digital literacy, and established virtual learning spaces to connect students and teachers. Joint planning and collaboration by all stakeholders, including students, education providers and health facilities, is now needed, with

Midwives' association

TABLE 3.3

Percentage of 78 countries in which midwives are authorized to provide contraceptive products, by WHO region and World Bank income group, 2019–2020

	Number of countries reporting	Contraceptive pills (%)	Contraceptive injections (%)	Emergency contraception (%)	Intrauterine devices (%)	Contraceptive implants (%)
WHO REGION						
Africa	29/47	100%	100%	100%	97%	100%
Americas	11/35	100%	100%	91%	100%	91%
Eastern Mediterranean	7/21	71%	71%	43%	57%	57%
Europe	13/53	54%	46%	46%	38%	23%
South-East Asia	7/11	100%	100%	100%	100%	71%
Western Pacific	11/27	91%	91%	91%	91%	91%
INCOME GROUP						
High	18/61	61%	56%	44%	50%	50%
Upper middle	12/55	83%	83%	83%	75%	75%
Lower middle	28/49	100%	100%	100%	100%	89%
Low	20/29	100%	100%	95%	95%	90%
TOTAL	**78/194**	**88%**	**87%**	**83%**	**83%**	**78%**

Source: ICM survey.

> **Midwives should be involved in SRMNAH decision-making at all levels including: Ministry of Health, health facilities, education institutions, regulatory authorities, research programmes, development projects.**
>
> *Midwives' association*

clear communications to reduce confusion and anxiety *(72)*.

Midway through 2020, ICM launched a global Covid-19 survey to determine the role of midwives' associations in response to the pandemic's impact on the midwives they represent. By December 2020, over half of the ICM member associations had responded. They reported high levels of stress and burnout among midwives, and most (70%) reported that midwives had experienced a lack or shortage of personal protective equipment (PPE). Associations reported that midwives had resourcefully addressed this situation by making their own PPE (43%), purchasing their own (53%), or improvising with whatever was available (48%). Some associations reported that midwives had reused

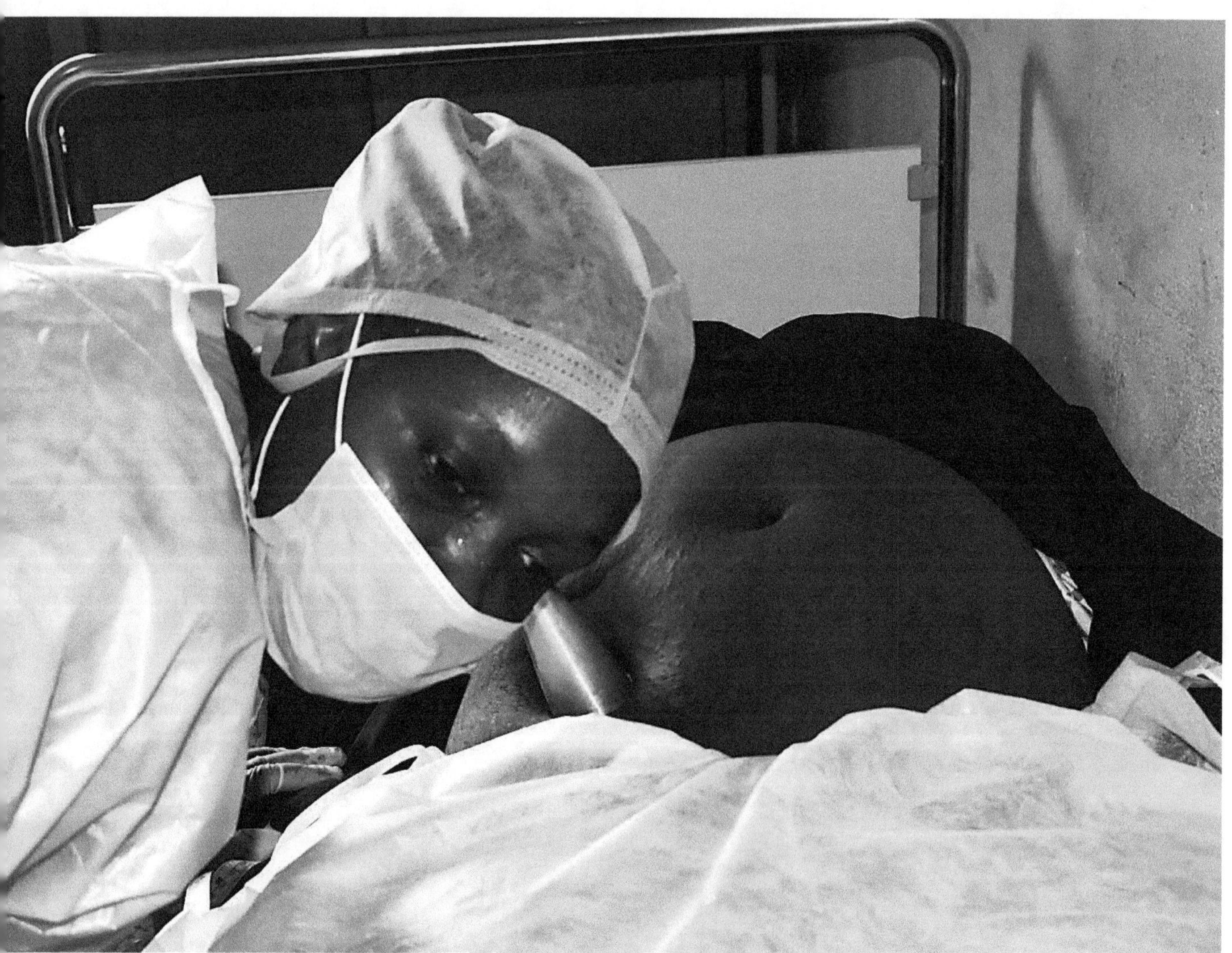

Midwife conducts antenatal check. © UNFPA Guinea.

Identifying and addressing the needs of midwives during Covid-19 in Latin America and the Caribbean

Early in 2020, it became clear that Covid-19 would have a major impact on UNFPA's plans for strengthening midwifery. To guide its response, the Latin America and the Caribbean Regional Office undertook an online survey of midwives to explore the pandemic's impact on their work and identify the support they needed to respond effectively. Over 1,000 responses were received from 12 countries. Over half of respondents thought they had not been adequately consulted or considered in their workplace's decision-making processes, and that there was insufficient PPE.

UNFPA developed a template for documenting innovative adjustments to service delivery and invited the presidents of professional midwives' associations to submit a summary of their practices using the template. Examples were shared by 23 midwives from 11 countries, including: using virtual technologies to maintain essential services, multidisciplinary efforts (including community outreach) in diverse settings to meet SRMNAH needs within a human rights framework, and the empowerment of midwives' associations and midwife leaders to work with politicians and health service leaders.

Videoconferences were held two to four times per month with midwives' association leaders, UNFPA staff and the ICM regional representative in Latin America. The agenda included sharing of statistics on Covid-19 infections and deaths. ICM member associations in Latin America prepared a declaration for the attention of Ministers of Health, highlighting the risks to mothers, newborns and families during the pandemic, and the need for PPE for midwives (73).

Restrictions relating to Covid-19 made it essential to find new ways to continue education and training for midwives. The University of Chile led the development and dissemination of Spanish-language resources for continuing education (74, 75). There is a regularly updated repository of information on Covid-19, including national guidelines, protocols, epidemiological information, and other materials designed to support midwifery work (76). UNFPA's Sub-Regional Office for the Caribbean provided a grant to the Caribbean Regional Midwives Associations for activities, including the development of a virtual continuing professional development programme (77). The topics, chosen in consultation with midwives, have included: mental health of midwives and mothers; continuity of sexual and reproductive health services during Covid-19; infection prevention and control during Covid-19; and respectful maternity care during Covid-19.

Contributed by Alma Virginia Camacho-Hübner (UNFPA Latin America and the Caribbean Regional Office).

---

single-use PPE (30%), worked without (26%) or just not attended work (7%).

Over half (54%) of responding associations reported that midwifery education courses had been closed in their countries, 90% of courses had changed to online learning and 25% to small group learning. Only 50% of those associations felt that students had access to practice areas or clinical placements some of the time, while 25% had no access. Almost two thirds (61%) of responding associations reported delays in midwifery students completing their studies.

One of the more positive reported effects of Covid-19 was improved collaboration between health professionals. Of the associations who responded to this question, 90% reported improved and positive collaborations between health professionals, who joined forces in different ways to help each other, including obstetricians, paediatricians, infection control specialists, nurses and in some cases the medical corps of defence units.

Midwives in many countries have made specific efforts to address the Covid-19 challenges in their own countries. Box 3.4 describes the work done in one UNFPA region to fully understand the needs of midwives as they continue to work through the pandemic. Box 3.5 highlights the key roles played by young midwife leaders in Malawi and Namibia.

Midwives contribute to national Covid-19 responses in Malawi and Namibia

Three participants in the ICM Young Midwife Leaders programme shared their experiences of strengthening their countries' response to the Covid-19 pandemic. In Malawi, the midwife leader conducted a situation analysis of how the pandemic was affecting midwives and their work and designed responses to the challenges identified. In Namibia, one leader contributed to the drafting of national policies and guidelines on caring for women with Covid-19 during pregnancy, childbirth and the postnatal period, and another contributed to the national committee on infection prevention and control.

The experiences of the three midwifery leaders showed: **Involving front-line SRMNAH workers leads to better decisions.** Those who work directly with service users bring a vital perspective to the decision-making process. Their contributions are often underestimated because of a perception that health workers lack planning and organizational skills. However, their input can prevent poor decision-making. For example, stopping a neonatal intensive care unit from being converted into a Covid-19 centre and relocating it further away from the labour ward; raising awareness that a national shortage of cord clamps, caused by diverting resources to Covid-19, was putting newborn lives at risk.

Midwives bring a unique perspective. Midwives' focus and passion relates specifically to SRMNAH, so their involvement at the highest level helps to ensure that the needs of SRMNAH service users and providers are not overlooked in the Covid-19 response. For example, ensuring that supplies of PPE are allocated fairly between and within health facilities; recognizing the fear felt by midwives working in health facilities and using this to design guidelines that communicate clearly and provide reassurance.

Networking enables midwives to take a seat at the table. Initially, no midwives were invited to contribute to Malawi's and Namibia's Covid-19 response. The support they received from ICM and their mentors through the Young Midwife Leaders programme empowered these three women to put themselves forward and make sure that midwives' voices were heard.

Contributed by Sylvia Hamata, Tekla Shiindi-Mbidi and Luseshelo Simwinga, with the support of Ann Yates (ICM).

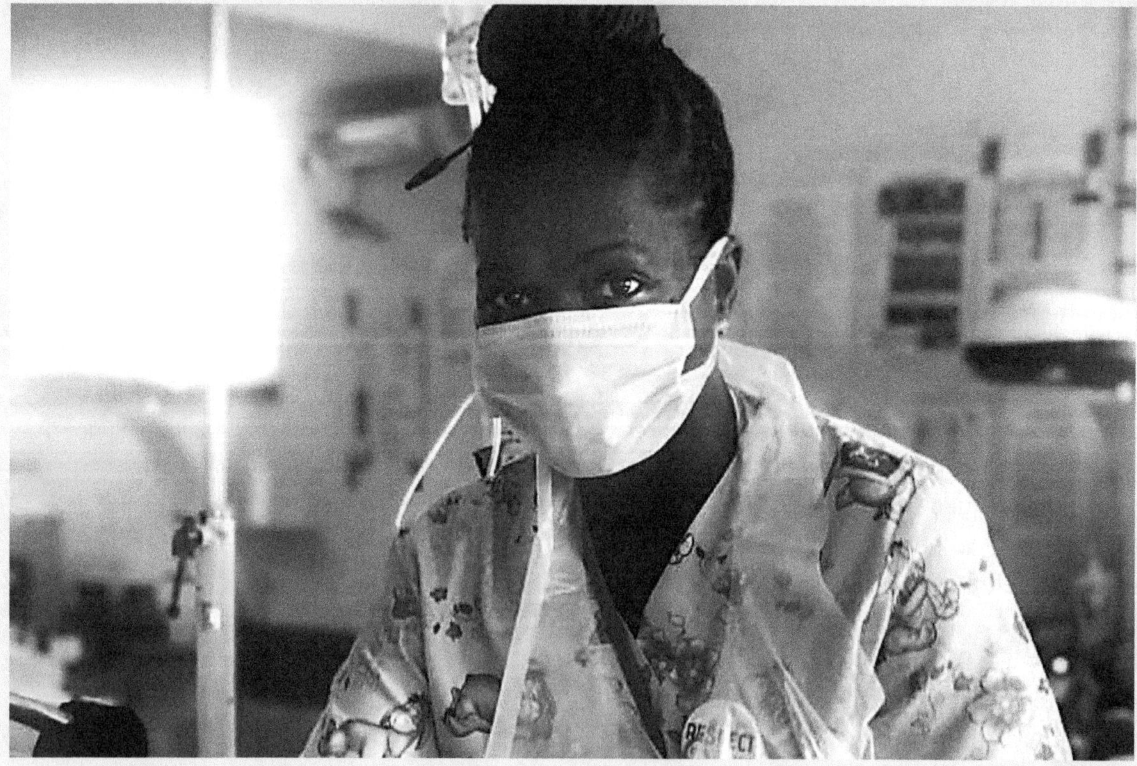

Luseshelo at work in Blantyre, Malawi. © White Ribbon Alliance.

NEED FOR AND AVAILABILITY OF MIDWIVES AND OTHER SRMNAH WORKERS

This chapter assesses the state of the world's SRMNAH workforce in 2019, and uses modelling to predict how this might change by 2030. The composition of the SRMNAH workforces varies: different countries use different job titles to describe occupations, and the roles and responsibilities of an occupation may differ between countries using the same job title. This variation in classification and nomenclature frustrates efforts to conduct national and global monitoring and analyses. For example, not all countries or languages distinguish clearly between midwives and other occupation groups, such as nurses, obstetricians and traditional birth attendants, and a midwife's scope of practice is not the same in every country. A recent review found 102 unique names used in low- and middle-income countries to describe health workers who attend births *(78)*. Similarly, not all countries adhere to the 2018 definition of skilled health personnel providing care during childbirth *(79)*.

The data shown in this chapter are mainly from NHWA (as at December 2020), as described in Chapter 1 and Webappendices 1–3. In addition to midwives, the analysis in this chapter includes other SRMNAH workers, in acknowledgement of the fact that an interdisciplinary team is necessary to meet the SRMNAH needs of all women, newborns and adolescents.

Data availability

All 194 WHO Member States were eligible for inclusion in SoWMy 2021, and all submitted at least one data item that is featured in this report. Effective workforce planning depends on the availability of high-quality data about both the

workforce and the pipeline that feeds it. The routine collection of a minimum set of data is essential (SoWMy 2014 listed 10 essential data items *(24)*) yet no country provided all these data items for all SRMNAH occupation groups. Box 4.1 describes the challenges for workforce data collection, and how these are being addressed in one WHO region.

In NHWA there was good availability of headcounts for midwives, nurses and doctors, and reasonably good availability of graduate numbers for midwives and nurses. Beyond these, data availability was limited, which restricts the scope for detailed analysis. The analysis and the accompanying country profiles rely heavily on imputed values, made necessary by missing data (see Webappendix 3).

The analysis in this chapter uses three key concepts to measure workforce availability and

---

KEY MESSAGES

▸ With its current composition and distribution, the world's SRMNAH workforce cannot meet the global need for essential SRMNAH care. There are shortages of all SRMNAH workers, especially of midwives.

▸ The biggest shortages are in low-income countries, especially in the WHO African Region.

▸ At the current rate of progress, by 2030 things will have improved only slightly, and most of the improvement will be in middle-income countries. The gap between high- and low-income countries is projected to widen.

accessibility: the number of health workers needed to provide essential services ("need"), the availability of health workers ("supply") and countries' capacity to employ them ("demand"). Each piece of analysis is based on a different number of countries, reflecting the differing levels of data availability for individual indicators. Each table and figure shows the number of reporting countries; Webappendix 4 shows which countries provided data for each piece of analysis. Where the number of reporting countries for a particular indicator is low, firm conclusions cannot be drawn. Further, analysis by region and income group may mask within-region and within-income group variations. The country profiles present individual country data.

SoWMy 2021 uses data collection methods different from those used in previous SoWMy reports, and defines occupation groups differently. For example, some countries that previously reported having professional midwives now report that their midwives are associate professionals. **While this represents progress in terms of acknowledging the importance of defining occupation groups consistently, it means that for many countries the data in SoWMy 2021 should not be directly compared with the data in earlier SoWMy reports**.

The need for SRMNAH workers

In this report, the **need** for SRMNAH workers is defined as the amount of SRMNAH worker time that would be required to achieve universal, high-quality coverage of the essential SRMNAH interventions listed in Webappendix 5 and taken from the *Global Strategy for Women's, Children's and Adolescents' Health (9)*. SoWMy 2014 used a similar definition, but a different list of essential interventions. This also affects comparability

---

BOX 4.1

The challenges of data collection and how these are being addressed in South-East Asia

Tracking progress on health workforce development can be challenging when only weak national data are available, and data collection can be a burdensome task for countries. Even before the Covid-19 pandemic, data collection and collation capacity were stretched in many countries due to competing needs, potentially undermining the quantity and quality of data reported to NHWA.

In 2014, WHO South-East Asia Region Member States made a commitment to a Decade for Health Workforce Strengthening. Its first review in 2016 found that lack of standard indicators and incomplete data were significant barriers to reporting on progress. For example, headcount data commonly come from health council registers, which can differ significantly from other data sources, such as census or health facility surveys, which are designed for different purposes.

With these challenges in mind, Member States in the Region agreed on 14 priority indicators to report via NHWA and to review progress in 2018 *(80)*. In the data collection for the *State of the World's Nursing 2020* report and this report, WHO Regional Office for South-East Asia and country offices built on this approach, coordinating across departments to minimize duplication of effort and to streamline communications with national government counterparts. Within countries, technical working groups, consisting of NHWA focal points and representatives from various stakeholders, such as health councils and education institutions, have played a critical role in triangulating various data sources, and agreeing on uniform data for submission to NHWA. This process led directly to greater ownership and better utilization of the data collected by countries.

Contributed by Masahiro Zakoji, Ai Tanimizu and Malin Bogren (WHO Regional Office for South-East Asia).

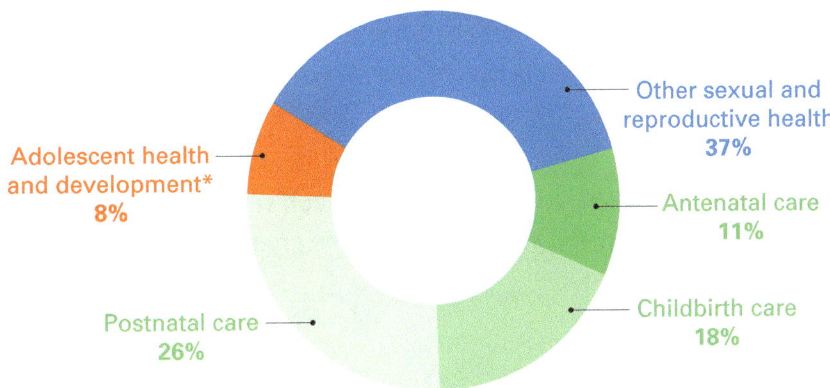

* The needs of adolescent girls aged 15–19 were included within those of women of reproductive age, so the estimate for adolescent health and development covers the sexual and reproductive health needs of girls aged 10–14 and boys aged 10–19.

Source: Estimates made for this report.

between SoWMy 2014 and SoWMy 2021: the need identified is higher in SoWMy 2021 due to its use of a more comprehensive list of essential interventions in the definition of need.

Globally, 6.5 billion SRMNAH worker hours would have been required to meet all the need in 2019. This is projected to increase to 6.8 billion hours by 2030. Figure 4.1 shows that 55% of the global need for health worker time for essential SRMNAH care is for maternal and newborn health interventions (antenatal, childbirth and postnatal care), 37% is for other sexual and reproductive health interventions such as counselling, contraceptive services, comprehensive abortion care, and detection and management of sexually transmitted infections, and 8% is for adolescent sexual and reproductive health interventions. The amount of time needed for postnatal care is more than double the time needed for antenatal care. This is mainly because postnatal care is needed for two people: in the first 24–48 hours postpartum, new mothers and newborns should both receive frequent interventions, which are more time-consuming than antenatal care visits. Also, some essential postnatal care interventions, although less common, are very time-consuming, e.g. caring for small and sick newborns and women with severe morbidities.

The two main drivers of need for SRMNAH workers are population size and fertility rate (81). Variations in these two factors mean that the need for SRMNAH workers is relatively high in the South-East Asia and African regions (1.6 billion and 1.5 billion hours respectively in 2019). Variations in fertility rates also influence the skill mix needed within the SRMNAH workforce: the workforce in high-fertility settings should contain a higher percentage of SRMNAH workers competent to provide maternal and newborn health care. For example, in the African region, over 60% of the SRMNAH worker time needed in 2019 was for maternal and newborn health interventions

> **KEY FINDINGS**
>
> ▸ Globally, 6.5 billion SRMNAH worker hours would have been required to meet all the need in 2019. This is projected to increase to 6.8 billion hours by 2030.
>
> ▸ Just over half (55%) of the global need for health worker time for essential SRMNAH care is for maternal and newborn health interventions (antenatal, childbirth and postnatal care), 37% is for other sexual and reproductive health interventions such as counselling, contraceptive services, comprehensive abortion care, and detection and management of sexually transmitted infections, and 8% is for adolescent sexual and reproductive health interventions.

(represented by the green segments in Figure 4.2), compared with 45% in the European and Western Pacific regions. As a result, although a relatively low **percentage** of the need in Africa is for "other sexual and reproductive health", this is still a large number

of hours: 375 million hours out of the region's total need for 1.5 billion hours. In absolute terms, this is similar to the 330 million hours needed in the Americas, but because the total amount of need in the Americas (750 million hours) is much lower than

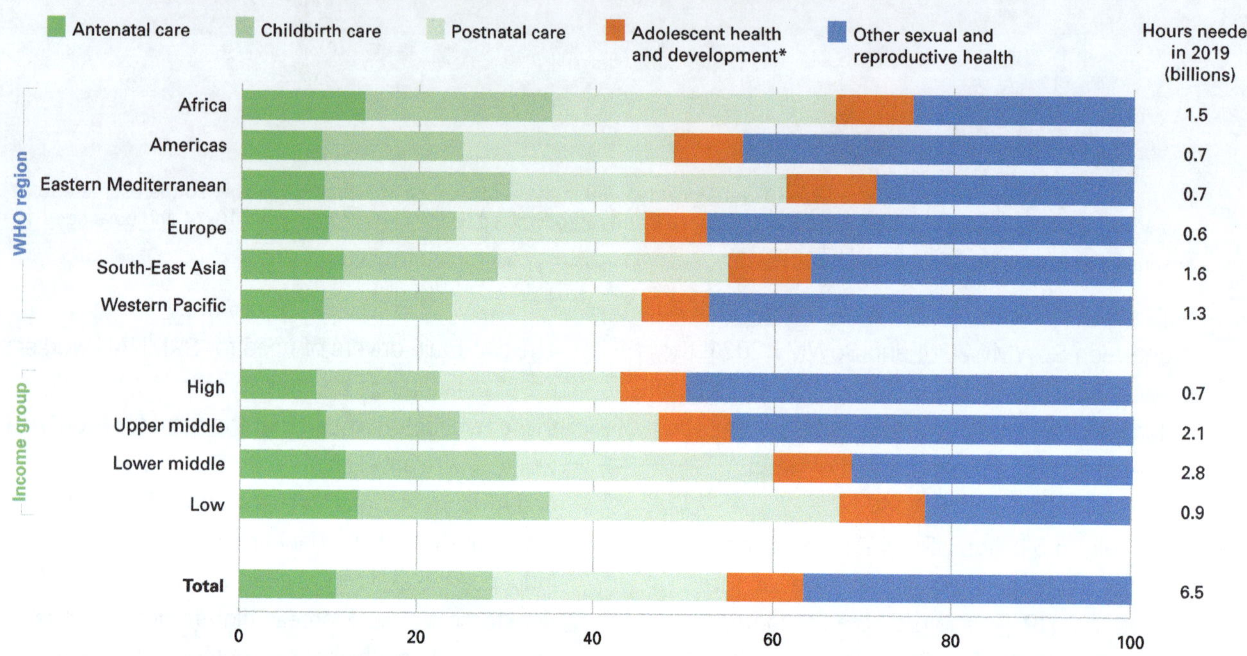

Figure 4.2 **Percentage of SRMNAH worker time needed at each stage in the continuum of care, 189 countries, by WHO region and World Bank income group, 2019**

* The needs of girls aged 15–19 are included in those of women of reproductive age, so the estimate for adolescent health and development covers the sexual and reproductive health needs of girls aged 10–14 and boys aged 10–19.

Source: Estimates made for this report.

in Africa, 330 million hours is a larger percentage of the total time needed.

Figures 4.1 and 4.2 present estimates of the amount of SRMNAH worker time **needed** at each stage of the continuum of care to achieve universal coverage: these figures do not represent the amount of time **actually devoted** to each stage. In many countries, postnatal care coverage is much lower than antenatal care coverage *(82)*. In those countries, the SRMNAH workforce may devote more of its available time to antenatal care than to postnatal care even though the amount of time needed for postnatal care is greater, leading to more unmet need for postnatal care than for antenatal care.

If available in sufficient numbers, and if fully educated, regulated and integrated within an interdisciplinary team, midwives could meet about 90% of the global need for essential SRMNAH interventions (see Webappendices 3 and 5).

Current SRMNAH workforce availability, composition and distribution

The 192 participating countries reported the number of SRMNAH workers using the occupation group definitions shown in Webappendix 1. Table 4.1 shows the total numbers reported. Very few countries reported headcounts for all SRMNAH occupation groups.[3] In particular, few countries provided headcounts for paramedical practitioners,

3 A small number of reporting countries does not necessarily indicate missing data: we do not expect all countries to report for all occupation groups. Some countries may not have that occupation group as part of their health workforce

▶ With its current composition and distribution, the world's SRMNAH workforce could meet 75% of the world's need for essential SRMNAH care, but in low-income countries, the workforce could meet only 41% of the need. Potential to meet the need is lowest in the African and Eastern Mediterranean WHO regions.

▶ If educated, regulated and integrated within an interdisciplinary team, midwives could meet about 90% of the global need for essential SRMNAH interventions, yet they account for just 8% of the SRMNAH workforce.

▶ There is a global needs-based shortage of 1.1 million "dedicated SRMNAH equivalent" (DSE) workers. This total number represents shortages in of all types of SRMNAH workers, but the largest shortage is of midwives and the wider midwifery workforce.

▶ Factors preventing the workforce from meeting all of the need include: insufficient numbers, inefficient skill mix, inequitable distribution, poor-quality education and training (including supervision and mentoring) and poor-quality regulation, which lead to poor quality of care (including disrespect and abuse) and poor SRMNAH outcomes.

▶ Covid-19 has reduced workforce availability. Access to SRMNAH services needs to be prioritized, and provided in a safe environment, despite the pandemic. SRMNAH workers need protection from infection, support to cope with stress and trauma, and creative/innovative solutions to the challenges of providing high-quality education and services.

TABLE 4.1

Number (thousands) of SRMNAH workers in 192 countries, 2019 (or latest available year since 2014)

Occupation group	Number of reporting countries	Number of workers reported (thousands)
Midwifery professionals	77	650.9
Midwifery associate professionals	22	477.3
Midwives not further defined	68	420.9
Nursing professionals	144	19,766.5
Nursing associate professionals	93	5317.9
Nurses not further defined	56	2386.2
Obstetricians and gynaecologists	191	532.7
Paediatrician practitioners	185	537.5
General medical practitioners	190	4109.9
Paramedical practitioners	40	345.0
Medical assistants	18	104.7
Community health workers	43	1950.9

Note: Many countries submitted a total headcount for all medical doctors, without providing headcounts for specialty (e.g. obstetrics, paediatrics). For these countries, assumptions were made about the proportion of medical doctors in each of the three medical doctor occupation groups in this table (see Webappendix 3).

Source: NHWA, 2020 update.

medical assistants and community health workers. For this reason, no analysis of these three occupation groups is included in this chapter, but they are shown in individual country profiles and are considered when estimating the potential of the SRMNAH workforce to meet the need.

Not all countries have the health care occupation group "midwives". Some rely on nurses with additional and specialized training in midwifery. To reflect this heterogeneity in occupations involved in providing midwifery care, SoWMy 2021 uses the term "wider midwifery workforce" which includes nurses with midwifery training, sometimes called "nurse-midwives". The grouping together of these nurses with midwives is not meant to imply that all members of this group work as midwives: it simply means that they have received a level of education or training in midwifery which qualifies them to practise as part of the wider midwifery workforce in their country. The available data do not indicate how many are working as midwives, how many as nurses, and how many as both.

The remaining analyses in this chapter use the following groupings of SRMNAH workers:

Wider midwifery workforce: including all professional and associate professional midwives, "midwives not further defined", and nurses (professional or associate) with midwifery training, hereafter called "nurse-midwives"

Nursing workforce excluding those with midwifery training: including all professional and associate professional nurses and "nurses not further defined", and excluding any nurses with midwifery training

SRMNAH doctors: including general medical practitioners, obstetricians/gynaecologists and paediatricians.

Current availability of the wider midwifery workforce

Headcounts for the wider midwifery workforce were available for 160 countries. These countries' data indicate a wider midwifery workforce of 1.9 million: an average density of 4.4 per 10,000 population (Table 4.2). Density is relatively high in the Western Pacific Region (5.9 per 10,000 population). It is higher in high- and middle-income countries than in

---

TABLE 4.2

Size (thousands) and density of wider midwifery workforce in 160 countries, by WHO region and World Bank income group, 2019 (or latest available year since 2014)

	Number of countries reporting headcount/all WHO Member States	Size of wider midwifery workforce* in thousands (% of global total)	Density per 10,000 population**
WHO REGION			
Africa	37/47 (79%)	259 (14%)	2.6
Americas	23/35 (66%)	160 (8%)	1.9
Eastern Mediterranean	15/21 (71%)	175 (9%)	3.2
Europe	52/53 (98%)	424 (22%)	4.6
South-East Asia	8/11 (73%)	588 (31%)	10.4
Western Pacific	25/27 (93%)	289 (15%)	5.9
INCOME GROUP			
High	55/61 (90%)	435 (23%)	3.7
Upper middle	42/55 (76%)	795 (42%)	6.5
Lower middle	37/49 (76%)	566 (30%)	4.3
Low	26/29 (90%)	98 (5%)	1.6
TOTAL	**160/194 (82%)**	**1,894 (100%)**	**4.4**

* Includes midwifery professionals, midwifery associate professionals, nurse-midwives, associate nurse-midwives and midwives not further defined.

** Total headcount in all countries in a region/income group, expressed as a ratio of the total population of that region/income group.

Notes: Indonesia and the USA have major effects on regional and income group densities. Excluding Indonesia, the density for South-East Asia is 4.6 and for upper-middle-income countries it is 3.6. Excluding the USA, the density for the Americas is 2.8 and for high-income countries it is 4.9. Excluding both of these countries, the global average is 3.8 per 10,000 population.

Source: NHWA, 2020 update.

low-income countries. Over half of the wider midwifery workforce is in the South-East Asia and European regions, where the respective densities are 10.4 and 4.6 per 10,000 population. Some regional and income group averages are skewed by populous countries with atypical densities, most notably Indonesia (which reports a very large number of associate professional midwives) and the United States of America (which reports a very small wider midwifery workforce). The notes following Table 4.2 show the effect of excluding these two countries from the global, regional and income group averages.

The numbers in Table 4.2 cannot be directly compared with the numbers reported in earlier SoWMy reports, because the data in this report are based on a much larger number and more diverse range of countries, and the data collection method was different. For these reasons, only cautious conclusions may be drawn about changes over time. For example, of the 56 low- and middle-income countries that featured in both SoWMy 2021 and a previous SoWMy report, 24 have a clear upward trajectory for the density of the wider midwifery workforce, 16 have a clear downward trajectory, three show no major change and 13 show no clear pattern.

Of the 1.9 million members of the wider midwifery workforce in the reporting countries, 651,000 (34%) are categorized as midwifery professionals, 477,000 (25%) as midwifery associate professionals, 421,000 (22%) as "midwives not further defined", 285,000 (15%) as nurse-midwives and 60,000 (3%) as associate nurse-midwives. Before 2019, it was not possible to enter data in NHWA for nurse-midwives as a specific group, but now they can be specified as a subset of nurses. Countries reporting for years prior to 2019 probably counted them as nurses, so there may be more nurse-midwives than are reported here.

The large number of "midwives not defined" is of concern because their competencies are not known. For the analysis, they were reclassified as either professional or associate professionals, based on factors such as education duration and previous data reporting patterns (see

Figure 4.3 **Percentage of wider midwifery workforce in each occupation group in 161 countries, by WHO region and World Bank income group, 2019 (or latest available year since 2014)**

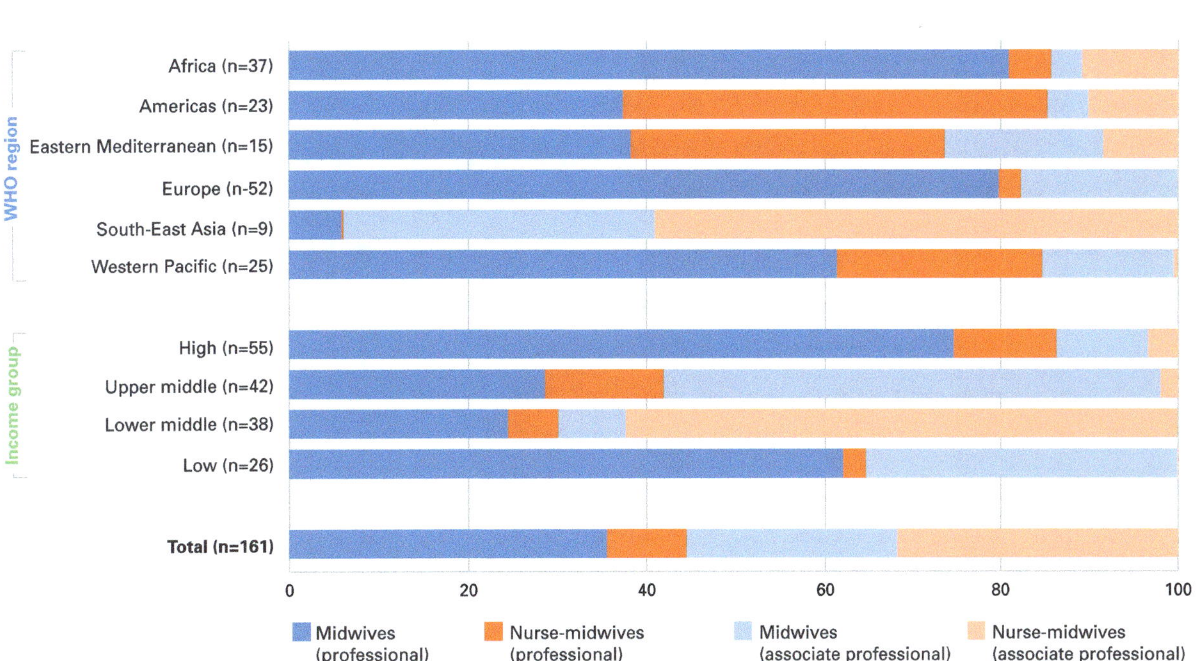

Note: This figure includes India, whereas Table 4.2 excludes India. This is because, as part of the reclassification process described in Webappendix 3, some of India's associate professional nurses were reclassified as associate professional nurse-midwives.

Source: NHWA, 2020 update, adjusted to compensate for large numbers of "midwives not defined".

Webappendix 3 for details). Based on these reclassified numbers, Figure 4.3 shows that South-East Asia is the only region with more associate professionals than professionals. The large population in this region has a pronounced effect on the global total, which shows slightly more associate professionals than professionals, even though in every other region there are more professionals than associates. Africa and Europe have the highest percentages of midwives; the Americas have the highest percentage of nurse-midwives. The wider midwifery workforce in high-income countries is mostly professionals, and to a lesser extent this is also true in low-income countries. In middle-income countries, most are associate professionals.

Current availability of other SRMNAH workers

Like all health-care professionals, the SRMNAH workforce is most effective when it operates within a fully enabled health system/work environment, with each member working to their full scope of practice, so that the team collectively possesses all the competencies required to provide high-quality, respectful SRMNAH care *(79)*. Availability of the wider midwifery workforce must therefore be considered in the context of availability of other key SRMNAH workers.

Analysis of the size and density of the nursing workforce (excluding nurse-midwives) and SRMNAH doctor workforces can be found in Webappendix 1. In addition to these indicators, it is important to consider how much of each occupation group's clinical time is available to spend on SRMNAH care: it would be inaccurate to assume that all SRMNAH workers spend all their available working time on SRMNAH. To address this issue, SoWMy 2021 uses the concept of a "dedicated SRMNAH equivalent" (DSE) worker. DSEs have been calculated using estimates about the average percentage of clinical contact time that each occupation group spends on SRMNAH (Webappendix 3).

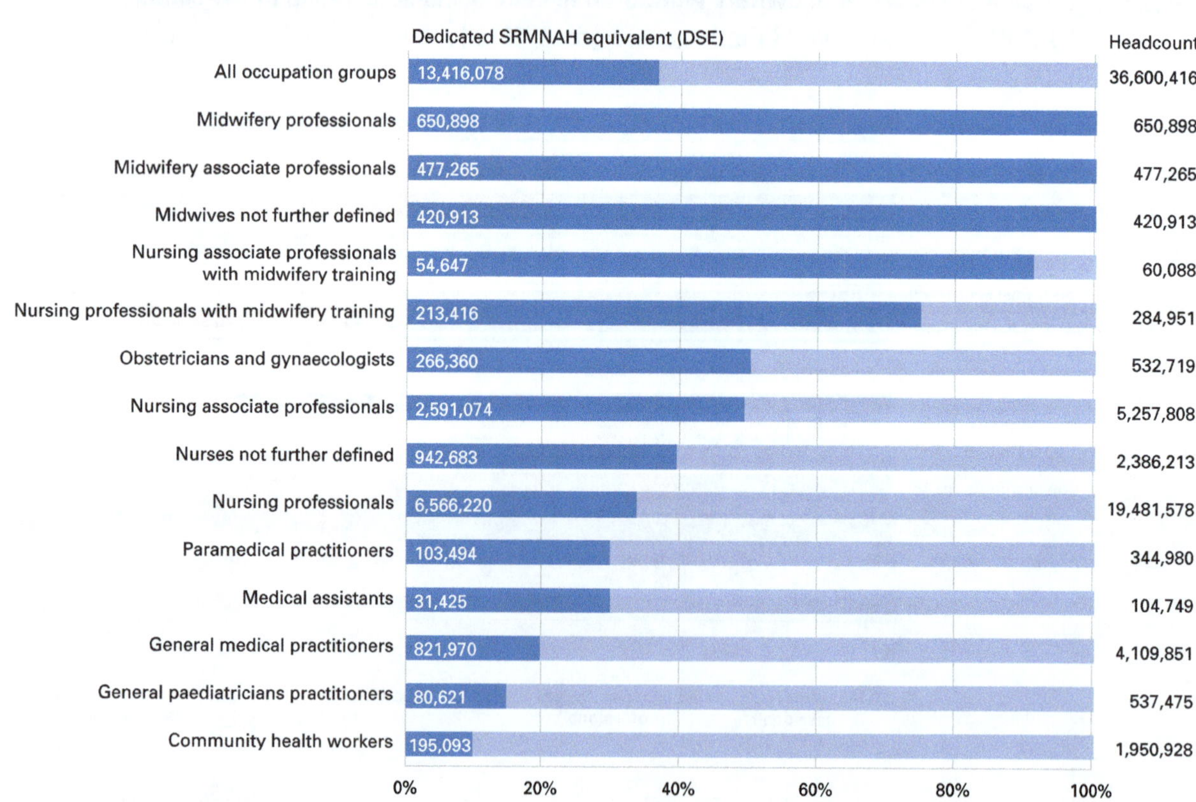

Figure 4.4 **SRMNAH workforce: headcount versus dedicated SRMNAH equivalent (DSE) in 192 countries, 2019 (or latest available year since 2014)**

Note: the "nursing professional" and "nursing associate professional" categories exclude nurses with midwifery training, who are shown separately.

Source: Headcounts from NHWA 2020 update. DSEs derived from headcounts and estimated % time spent on SRMNAH.

The impact of the DSE adjustment is illustrated in Figure 4.4: the DSE workforce is 13.4 million: 37% of the headcount of 36.6 million. Ideally, the DSE calculation would also take into account part-time working and the proportion of health workers who are clinically active. The DSE figures for countries with high rates of part-time working or large numbers of health workers in non-clinical roles will therefore over-estimate the amount of SRMNAH worker time available for the delivery of SRMNAH interventions.

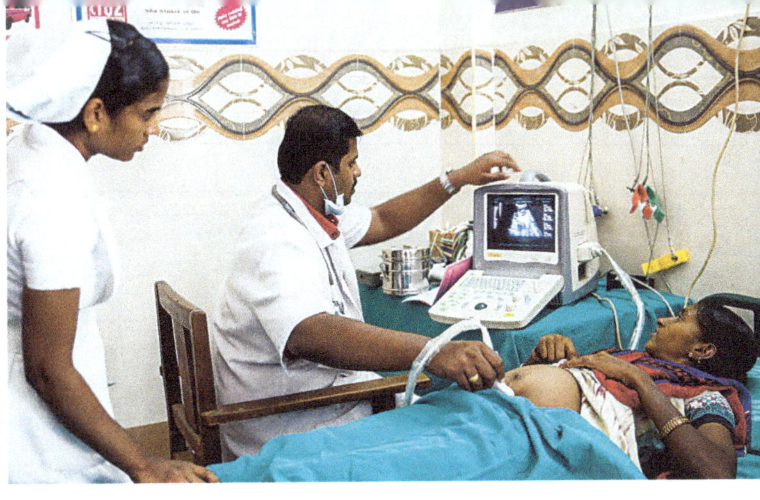
Ultrasound scanning at Urban Primary Health Centre in Lakshmipuram, Vellore, India. © Gates Archive/Mansi Midha.

Composition of SRMNAH workforce

Figure 4.5 shows the composition of the main occupation groups within the SRMNAH workforce in 192 reporting countries, in total, by WHO region and World Bank income group. These charts exclude SRMNAH workers other than midwives, nurses and doctors, due to lack of data.

By headcount, 77% of workers in the three key SRMNAH occupation types are nurses without midwifery training, 15% are SRMNAH doctors and 8% are members of the wider midwifery workforce. By DSE, 72% are nurses without midwifery training, 19% are members of the wider midwifery workforce and 9% are SRMNAH doctors, although there are variations by region and income group. The wider midwifery workforce accounts for a relatively large percentage of the DSE workforce in Africa and South-East Asia, the majority being

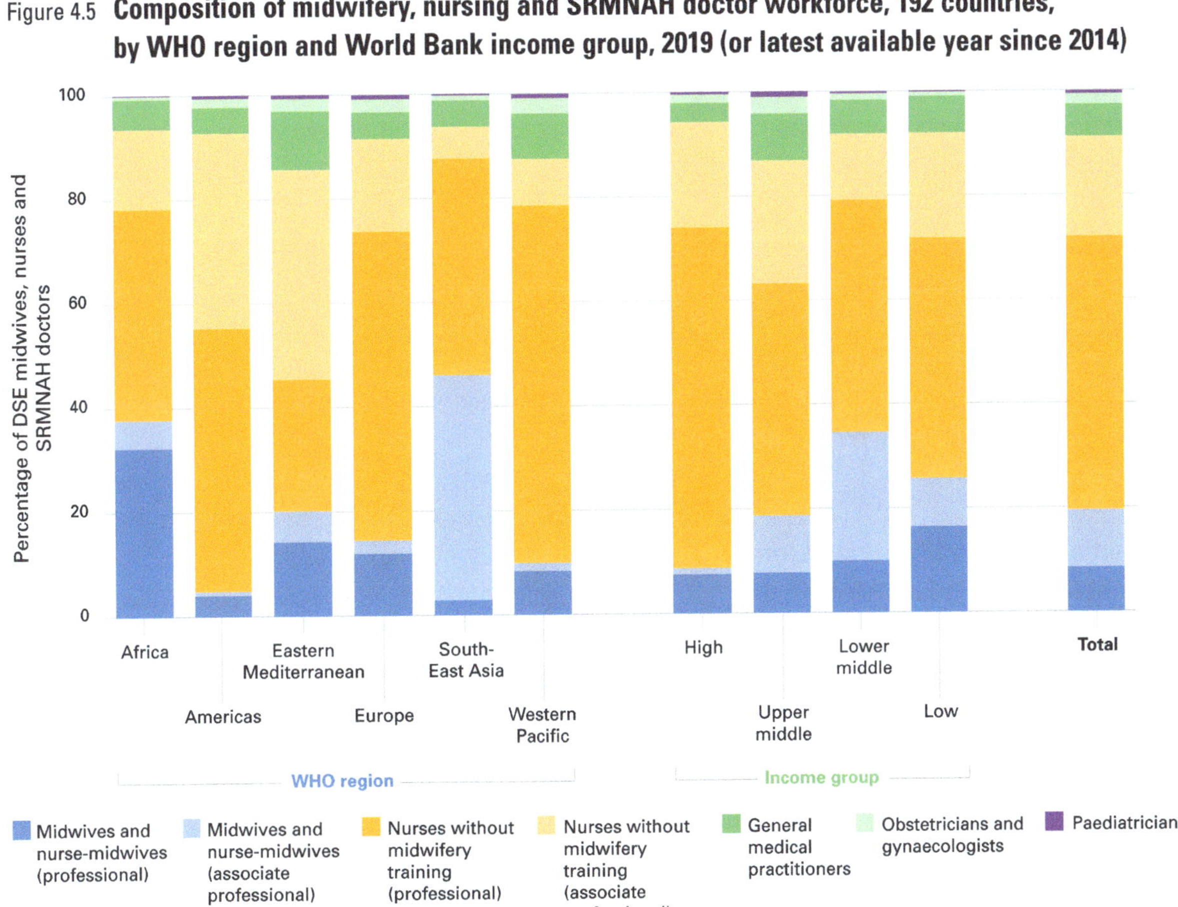

Figure 4.5 **Composition of midwifery, nursing and SRMNAH doctor workforce, 192 countries, by WHO region and World Bank income group, 2019 (or latest available year since 2014)**

Source: Headcounts from NHWA, 2020 update. DSEs derived from headcounts and estimated % time spent on SRMNAH.

Midwives' association

professionals in Africa and associate professionals in South-East Asia. In the Eastern Mediterranean Region, SRMNAH doctors account for a relatively large percentage of the DSE workforce. The wider midwifery workforce accounts for a relatively large percentage of the total in lower-middle- and low-income countries.

Although nearly all countries reported headcounts for doctors and nurses, only 160 reported headcounts for the wider midwifery workforce. This may be because the remaining 34 countries have no midwives, or because their numbers are not reported. If the latter, the wider midwifery workforce will account for a larger percentage of the global SRMNAH workforce than is shown in the chart. This may affect the Western Pacific Region more than others, because China's nurses and SRMNAH doctors are included, but China did not provide a midwife headcount.

Potential of the SRMNAH workforce to meet the need for essential interventions

The country profiles show estimates of "potential met need" (PMN): the extent to which the supply of DSE workers is large enough and has the appropriate skill mix to meet the need for essential SRMNAH interventions. Taking into account each country's demography and epidemiology, PMN estimates the maximum percentage of the need for essential SRMNAH interventions that could potentially be met by

the current workforce, *if it was well educated, equitably distributed and working within an enabling environment* (and thus able to deliver high-quality care). An enabling environment means that SRMNAH workers can practise to their full scope, are accountable for independent decisions within the regulated standard operating procedure, work within a functional health infrastructure with adequate human resources, equipment and supplies, have access to timely and respectful consultation, collaboration and referral, be safe from physical and emotional harm and have equitable compensation, including salary and working conditions.

Where constraints prevent the workforce from operating to its full potential (e.g. poor infrastructure, ineffective supply chains, high absenteeism, poor-quality education, inequitable geographical distribution) the actual level of need being met will be lower than is indicated by the PMN estimate.

The PMN estimates are based on assumptions about the clinical time needed to achieve universal coverage of the essential SRMNAH interventions (Webappendix 5) and about which SRMNAH occupation groups should be competent to perform which essential interventions (Webappendix 6). For this purpose, it was necessary to assign midwives and nurses "not further defined" to either the professional or associate professional occupation groups, according to the rules set out in Webappendix 3.

Individual country PMN estimates are shown in the country profiles for 157 countries with headcount data in NHWA for all three key SRMNAH occupation groups: wider midwifery workforce, nursing workforce without midwifery training and SRMNAH doctors. Table 4.3 shows regional and income group averages from these countries. The overall PMN for Europe and the Americas is close to 100%, whereas the overall PMN for Africa is just 51%. A clear pattern emerges by income group: the SRMNAH workforce could potentially meet 99% of the need in high-income countries, but just 41% of the need in low-income countries could be met by the current workforce.

A low PMN indicates that the SRMNAH workforce is too small and/or does not have the correct composition to meet the need. A high PMN indicates a workforce large enough to meet the need, but not necessarily with optimal composition. For example, a country with many midwives could achieve the same PMN as a country with many doctors, because the time required to deliver interventions is allocated to the available competent occupation groups. Thus, if there are few or no midwives in a workforce, the time required for interventions that could be delivered by a midwife is allocated to the available nurses or doctors. However, it could be argued that it is inefficient and expensive to routinely allocate to doctors tasks that could be performed by other competent occupation groups.

Furthermore, without the option to consult a midwife, women, newborns and adolescents are deprived of the unique philosophy of care that midwives provide.

It is therefore important to critically evaluate the **composition** of the SRMNAH workforce as well as its overall **size**. To that end, the country profiles also estimate the number of DSEs required for 100% PMN. These estimates are based on the allocation of tasks to a **preferred** occupation group. The preferred group was selected on the basis of the competencies it should have if properly educated and regulated (see Webappendix 6). Tasks are allocated to doctors last, on the premise that doctors (relatively expensive to educate and employ,

Potential met need estimates in 157 countries, by WHO region and World Bank income group, 2019 (or latest available year since 2014)

	Number of countries reporting headcount/all WHO Member States	Potential met need estimate	
		Mean*	Range**
WHO REGION			
Africa	36/47 (77%)	51%	8% - 100%
Americas	23/35 (66%)	95%	27% - 100%
Eastern Mediterranean	15/21 (71%)	69%	7% - 100%
Europe	49/53 (92%)	98%	74% - 100%
South-East Asia	9/11 (82%)	78%	57% - 100%
Western Pacific	25/27 (93%)	87%	32% - 100%
INCOME GROUP			
High	52/61 (85%)	99%	95% - 100%
Upper middle	42/55 (76%)	91%	56% - 100%
Lower middle	37/49 (76%)	73%	30% - 100%
Low	26/29 (90%)	41%	7% - 100%
TOTAL	**157/194 (81%)**	**75%**	**7% - 100%**

* The total amount of SRMNAH worker time needed in countries in that group divided by the total amount of time allocated in those countries (i.e. a weighted mean). Thus, if a country had more time available than needed, its "excess" time was excluded from the regional, income group and global estimates.

** This shows the lowest and the highest individual country estimate in that group (there is at least one country with 100% in every group).

Source: Headcounts from NHWA, 2020 update. Potential met need estimated by the method described in Webappendix 3.

and needed only if medical intervention is indicated) should only be the preferred occupation group if no other occupation group is competent to perform the task. If the PMN estimate is high but the "required" numbers are very different from the "forecast" numbers within an occupation group, this may indicate suboptimal composition of the SRMNAH workforce.

Allocating interventions to preferred occupation groups enables the needs-based shortage of different SRMNAH occupation groups to be estimated (Webappendix 3). This analysis is based on the 157 countries with data on the wider midwifery workforce, the nursing workforce excluding those with midwifery training and SRMNAH doctors. Not all these countries have a shortage, but those which do have a **total needs-based shortage of 1.1 million DSE midwives, nurses and SRMNAH doctors, 0.9 million DSE of which are midwives/nurse-midwives**. The worst shortage is in the WHO African Region, accounting for 56% of the total shortage. Most of the remaining shortages are in the Eastern Mediterranean and Americas regions.

Impact of Covid-19 on SRMNAH worker availability

The headcount data reported above predate the Covid-19 pandemic, whose impact on SRMNAH worker availability is still being evaluated. Some impacts will be temporary: e.g. a recent WHO survey noted that many disruptions to SRMNAH services were due to staff redeployment for Covid-19 relief (83), and there is evidence that this was sometimes due to SRMNAH care not being deemed essential (84). To address these temporary impacts, WHO issued interim guidance on health workforce policy and management in the context of Covid-19 (85). The pandemic will probably also have a lasting impact on health worker availability. Many countries lack robust data on the number of infected health workers, due to lack of formal reporting mechanisms, but emerging data indicate that health care workers are at increased risk of infection (86, 87). In the early stages of the pandemic, shortages of PPE may have contributed to this increased risk.

Although many questions remain unanswered, thousands of health workers are known to

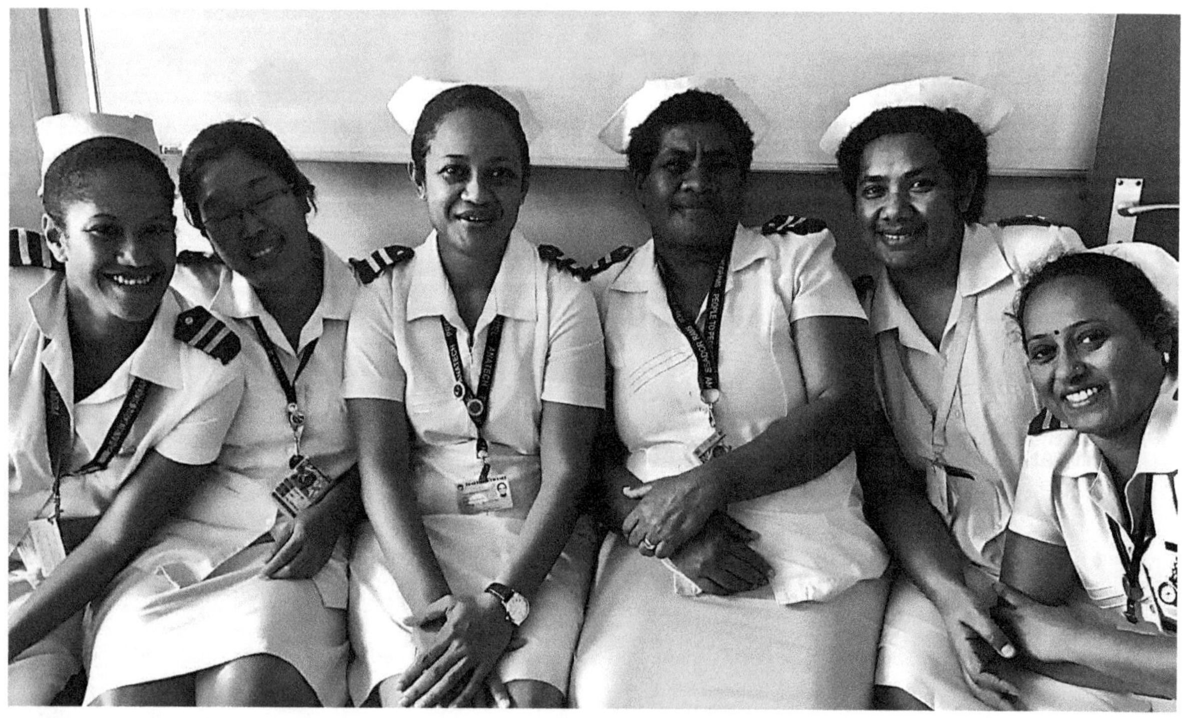

Nurses and midwives at Lautoka Hospital antenatal clinic, Fiji. © Felicity Copeland

have died *(88-90)*. Additionally, most national nursing associations (80%) have received reports of mental distress from nurses working in Covid-19 response, leading to concerns about burnout and traumatization *(90)*. Many countries have seen incidents of stress at work compounded by abuse and stigmatization from the public *(91)*. There are signs that this will lead to losses from the health workforce, exacerbating current and projected workforce shortages. ICM issued a global call to action to protect midwives from Covid-19 to enable them to continue providing essential care *(92)*.

There is an opportunity to build the health workforce back better through post-Covid-19 economic recovery plans *(93)*. With significant numbers of jobs lost due to the pandemic, in an already depleted global health workforce *(12)*, the future workforce could be strengthened by increasing education capacity and supporting individuals to retrain or transition into health care.

Future SRMNAH workforce availability

KEY FINDINGS

▸ At current rates, the SRMNAH workforce is projected to be capable of meeting 82% of the need by 2030: only a small improvement on the current 75%. The gap between low-income countries and high- and middle-income countries is projected to widen by 2030, increasing inequality.

▸ To close the gap by 2030, 1.3 million new DSE worker posts (mostly midwives/nurse-midwives, mostly in Africa) need to be created in the next 10 years. At current rates, only 0.3 million of these are expected to be created, leaving a projected shortage of 1 million by 2030.

▸ The need to step up the production and deployment of SRMNAH workers is not confined to countries with a needs-based shortage. Many countries (including some high-income countries) are forecast to have insufficient SRMNAH workers to meet demand by 2030.

Future supply

Effective workforce planning and management requires understanding why people join and leave the workforce, and how this will affect future workforce availability. Future availability is influenced by a number of factors, including domestic production of new graduates, international migration and the age profile of the workforce.

Fewer than half of WHO Member States provided NHWA data on domestic production of midwives and nurses, and even fewer provided these data about SRMNAH doctors. This makes it difficult to draw overall conclusions about whether the world, and individual regions and countries, are producing enough graduates to meet future need and demand. At country level, where graduate numbers were provided, they are shown in the country profile and were used to project workforce numbers to 2030. Otherwise, standard assumptions were applied when calculating these projections (see Webappendix 3).

Similarly, few countries provided data on international migration of SRMNAH workers. Among those who did, SRMNAH doctors and the nursing workforce (excluding those with midwifery training) were more likely than the wider midwifery workforce to be foreign-born or foreign-trained. This may reflect the relative diversity of midwife roles and education, which make midwives less easily "transferable" to a different country's health system. However, almost half of the countries reporting on the wider midwifery workforce were in the European Region, and over half were high-income countries, so these results cannot be generalized to other parts of the world. The low- and middle-income countries that did report on these indicators tended to report very small percentages of foreign-born and foreign-trained SRMNAH workers.

The age structure of the SRMNAH workforce is an important indicator of future availability: if more are approaching retirement age than are young, then it will be difficult to ensure sufficient availability in the near future. Many countries were unable to provide data about the age distribution of all their SRMNAH workers, but 75 did so for the wider midwifery workforce (as shown in the country profiles), 70 for SRMNAH doctors and 106 for the nursing workforce excluding those with midwifery training. The green line in Figure 4.6 represents equilibrium between the oldest and youngest age cohorts, the blue dots represent countries whose wider midwifery workforce contains more aged <35 than approaching retirement age, and the red dots represent countries with an ageing workforce (more approaching retirement age than aged <35). Most reporting countries are represented by blue dots, but 19 countries were identified as at risk of an ageing workforce. Similar analysis for SRMNAH doctors found 26 countries at risk of an ageing SRMNAH doctor workforce, and the *State of the World's Nursing 2020* report showed 18 countries at risk of an ageing nursing workforce *(16)*.

Half of the countries with an ageing wider midwifery workforce and one third of the countries with an ageing SRMNAH doctor workforce are high-income countries. Other than this, there are no clear patterns by region or income group: there are countries from every region and every income group both above and below the green line.

The SRMNAH workforces in the South-East Asia and Eastern Mediterranean regions have relatively young age profiles, especially for midwives, nurses and general medical practitioners. For obstetricians/gynaecologists and paediatricians, however, the youngest profile is in the African Region.

Very few countries, and no low-income countries, were able to provide data on the number of SRMNAH workers who chose to leave the workforce in the most recent year: eight coun-

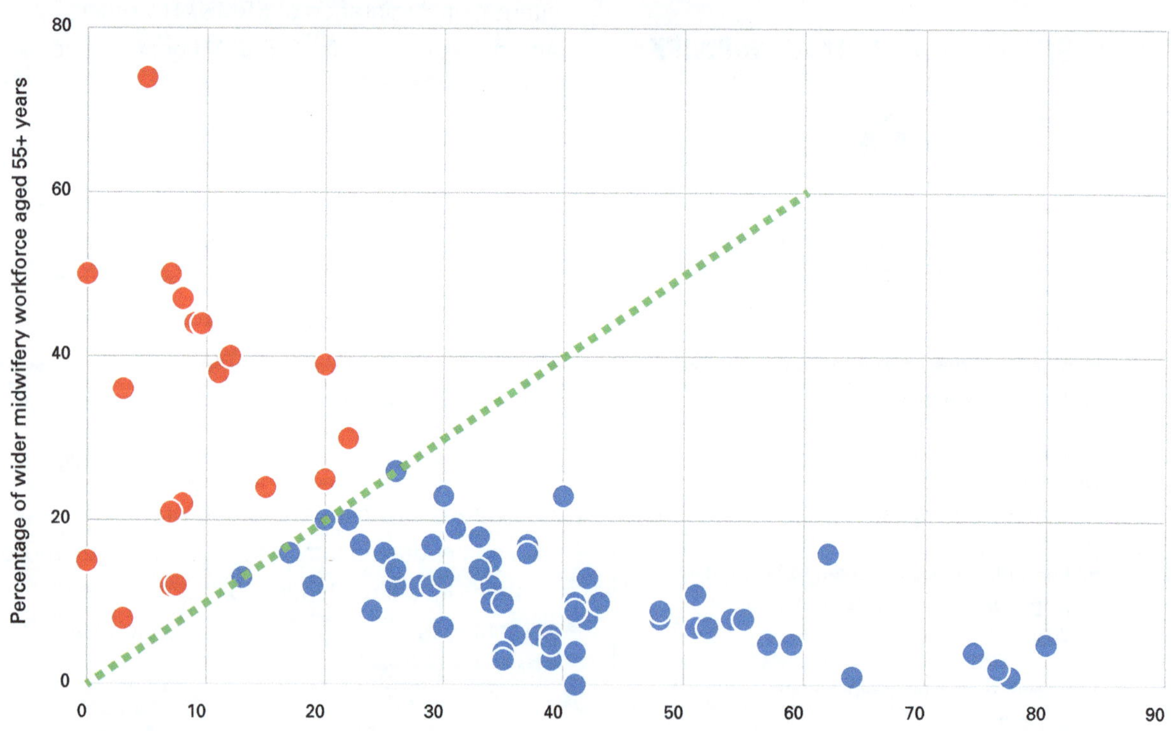

Figure 4.6 **Relative percentages of the wider midwifery workforce aged 55+ years and under 35 years, 75 countries, 2019 (or latest available year since 2014)**

Source: NHWA, 2020 update.

tries provided data about the wider midwifery workforce, 23 about the nursing workforce excluding those with midwifery training, and four about SRMNAH doctors. On average, these countries reported that 4% of their wider midwifery workforce, 9% of the nursing workforce (excluding those with midwifery training) and 5% of SRMNAH doctors chose to leave the national workforce in the most recent year. However, these averages mask wide variations between countries: for example, estimates of voluntary attrition from the wider midwifery workforce ranged from 1% to 22% of the current headcount. A high rate of attrition is unsustainable without a major annual influx of new graduates and/or in-migrants, and even with such an influx the loss of experienced workers may have implications for quality of care. The numbers of leavers, their reasons for leaving and their destinations are vital information which is often lacking (94).

Using the above data and evidence-based estimates when data are missing (see Webappendix 3) the country profiles project the SRMNAH workforce supply estimates to 2030. This analysis indicates that the supply of DSE workers will grow from 13.5 million in 2019 to 20.1 million in 2030 (a 49% increase).

Future need and the workforce's potential to meet that need

Having projected the supply to 2030, it is then compared with the projected need, yielding a 2030 PMN estimate. These projections indicate that, although most countries are on track to improve their PMN by 2030, many are projected to remain well short of 100%. In the 157 countries for which this analysis was possible, the average PMN is projected to increase from 75% in 2019 to 82% in 2030. Figure 4.7 shows that most of that improvement will be in middle-income countries. Some improvement is also projected

Figure 4.7   **Projected potential met need in 157 countries, by WHO region and World Bank income group, 2019, 2025 and 2030**

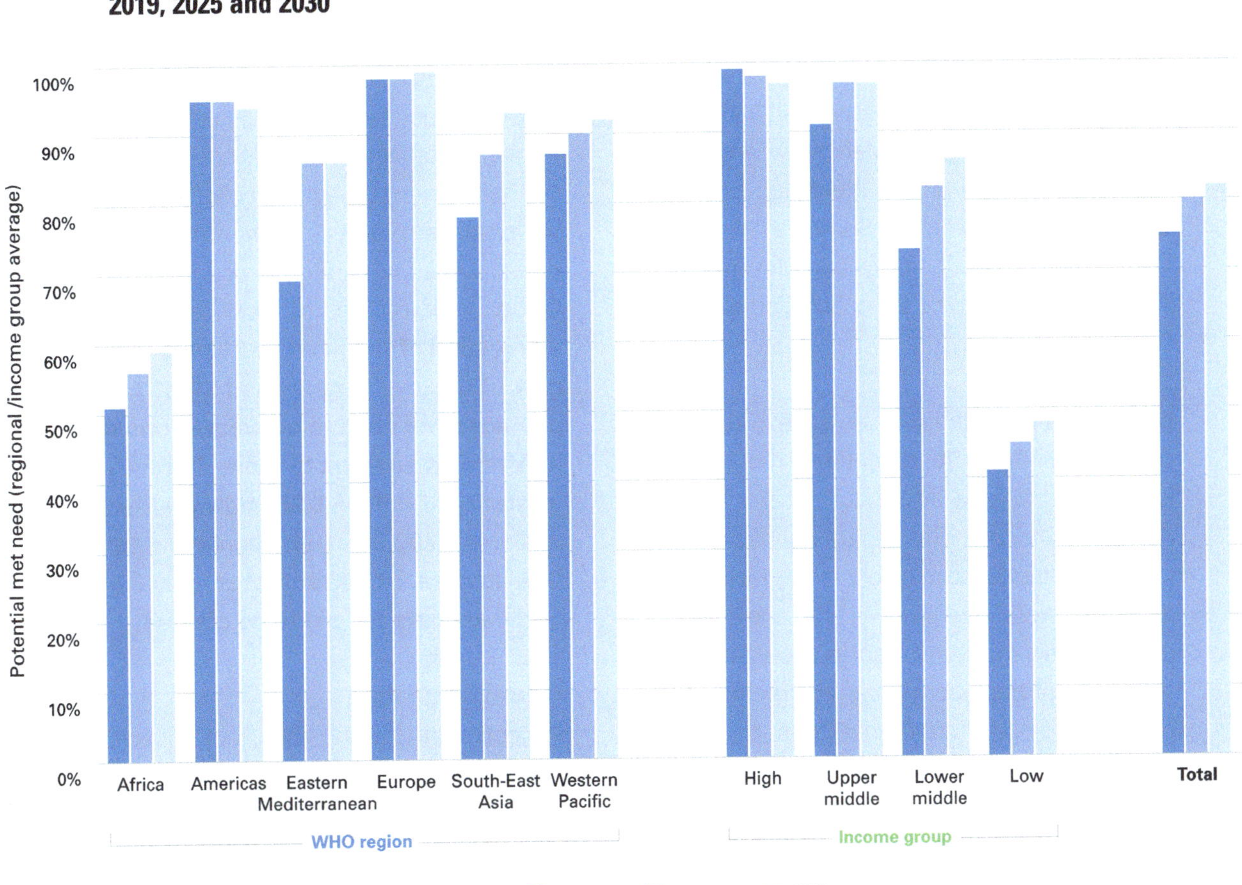

Source: Estimates made for this report.

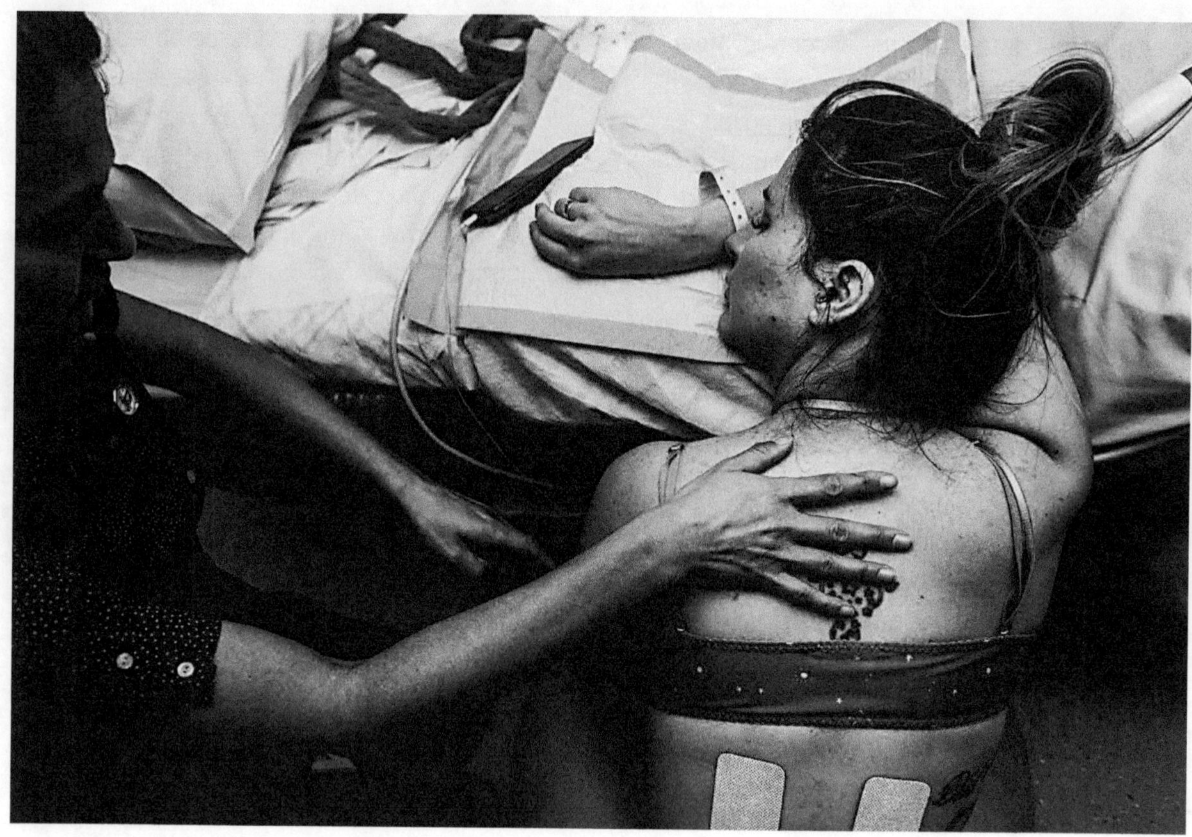

Midwife gives a calming touch. © Amber Grant.

for low-income countries, but the average PMN for low-income countries in 2030 will still be under 50%. It also shows that the regional average PMN is set to increase between 2019 and 2030 in all WHO regions except the Americas, where it is projected to remain at the current high level. The Eastern Mediterranean and South-East Asia regions are projected to see the biggest improvements. Africa is projected to be the only region with a PMN below 60% in 2030.

Despite the projected 49% increase in the size of the DSE workforce, its potential to meet the need is projected to grow by a much smaller amount (from 75% to 82%). This is partly because some countries already have a very high PMN, so their increased workforce size will not have a big effect on this measure. Also, in absolute terms, two thirds of the global workforce growth is projected to occur in the South-East Asia and Eastern Mediterranean regions, whereas most of the needs-based shortage is – and will remain – in the WHO African Region.

As stated above, there is a current shortage of 1.1 million DSEs, of which 900,000 are midwives. Projections to 2030 indicate that this shortage will decrease to 1 million DSEs, of which 750,000 will be midwives, with the most serious shortages still in the WHO African Region. In other words, if all countries continue on their current trajectory, collectively they will produce midwives, nurses and SRMNAH doctors at a faster rate than currently, but not fast enough to meet the growing global need. **To meet all of the need by 2030, 1.3 million new DSE midwife, nurse and SRMNAH doctor positions will need to be created (mostly in Africa) in addition to those currently in existence: 1 million DSE midwives/nurse-midwives, 200,000 DSE nurses and 100,000 DSE doctors. At current rates, only 0.3 million of these posts are set to be created.**

Future demand

Projecting the PMN is important, especially for countries with insufficient SRMNAH workers to meet the most basic SRMNAH needs. However, even countries with 100% PMN can have acknowledged shortages, because *demand* for SRMNAH workers and capacity to employ them may exceed needs-based thresholds. Projecting future unmet demand, as well as need, for the SRMNAH workforce is therefore essential for formulating workforce policy to prevent future mismatches.

SoWMy 2021 adopts an established labour market approach to project future demand for SRMNAH workers, using an economic model based on projected economic growth, demographics and health spending by both governments and individuals (95). Demand reflects the willingness of governments and other purchasers to pay for health care, which in turn drives demand for employing health workers.

The model starts with the assumption that all countries currently employ the number of SRMNAH workers that they can afford.[4] Then, by comparing the demand predicted in 2030 with the projected supply in that same year, projections of demand/supply mismatches are made for 2030. The results show that, by 2030, demand for DSE workers in 143 countries will rise and the overall PMD will be 92%, i.e. the supply will be 92% of what the countries can collectively afford to employ. In half of these countries (n=71), the model predicts that current supply projections will not keep pace with demand, resulting in a net demand-based shortage of just over one million DSEs. This overall picture masks substantial diversity between countries, with some projected to experience significant demand-based shortages (PMD below 50%) while in other countries supply will exceed demand, leading to surpluses (PMD above 105%). PMD below 50% will be more prevalent in low-income countries although, perhaps surprisingly, many high- and middle-income countries will also face moderate demand-based shortages (PMD 50%-95%) (Figure 4.8).

Figure 4.8 **Projected supply compared with projected demand in 143 countries, by WHO region and World Bank income group, 2030**

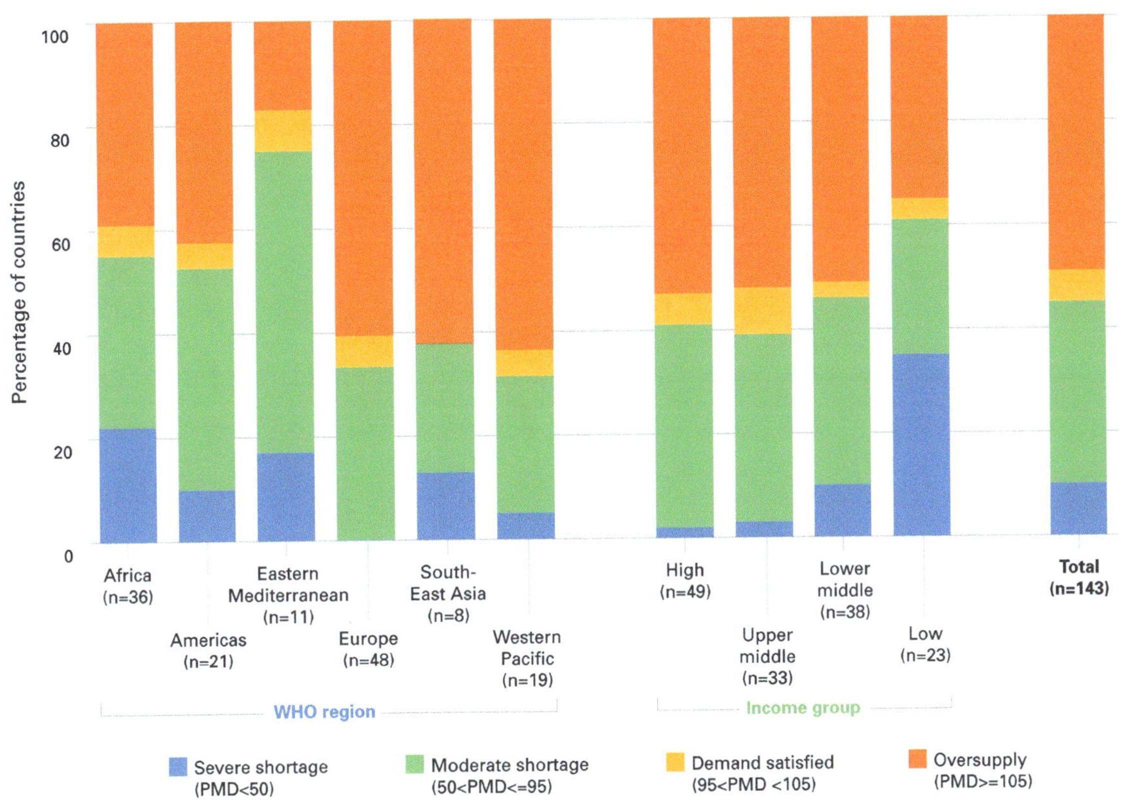

PMD = percentage met demand.

Source: Estimates made for this report.

4   This is unlikely to be true for all countries, but currently there is no established, standard method of estimating the number of unfilled posts.

Many low-income countries face low growth in both demand and supply, which are often both below what is needed to cover essential SRMNAH needs. Figure 4.9 plots PMN against PMD, with each dot representing a country, and the colours of the dots representing World Bank income group classifications. It shows that of 18 low- and lower-middle-income countries that face severe needs-based shortages (the bottom half of the graph), 15 will also have demand-based shortages (five moderate and 10 severe). In these countries, greater investments will be required to boost market-based demand and supply, and to align them more closely with population SRMNAH needs.

In contrast, the 35 countries facing a moderate needs-based shortage include 21 that are projected either to have satisfied their economic-based demand for workers or to have exhibited the paradox of surplus demand but a moderate needs-based shortage. This indicates that the countries' GDP growth and health spending are not forecast to keep pace with growing need for SRMNAH services due to increased population pressures. This is likely to lead to unemployed health workers. These are not only low-income countries, but also upper-middle- and high-income countries. A third of the countries with no needs-based shortage forecast (35 of 90), many of them in the high-income category, will need to significantly accelerate the pace of health worker production to ensure their supply of SRMNAH workers meets the demand. This could potentially raise the cost of health workers, stimulate labour movements across borders and lead to further inequalities.

Figure 4.9 **Projections of potential met need and percentage met demand for SRMNAH workforce in 143 countries, by World Bank income group, 2030**

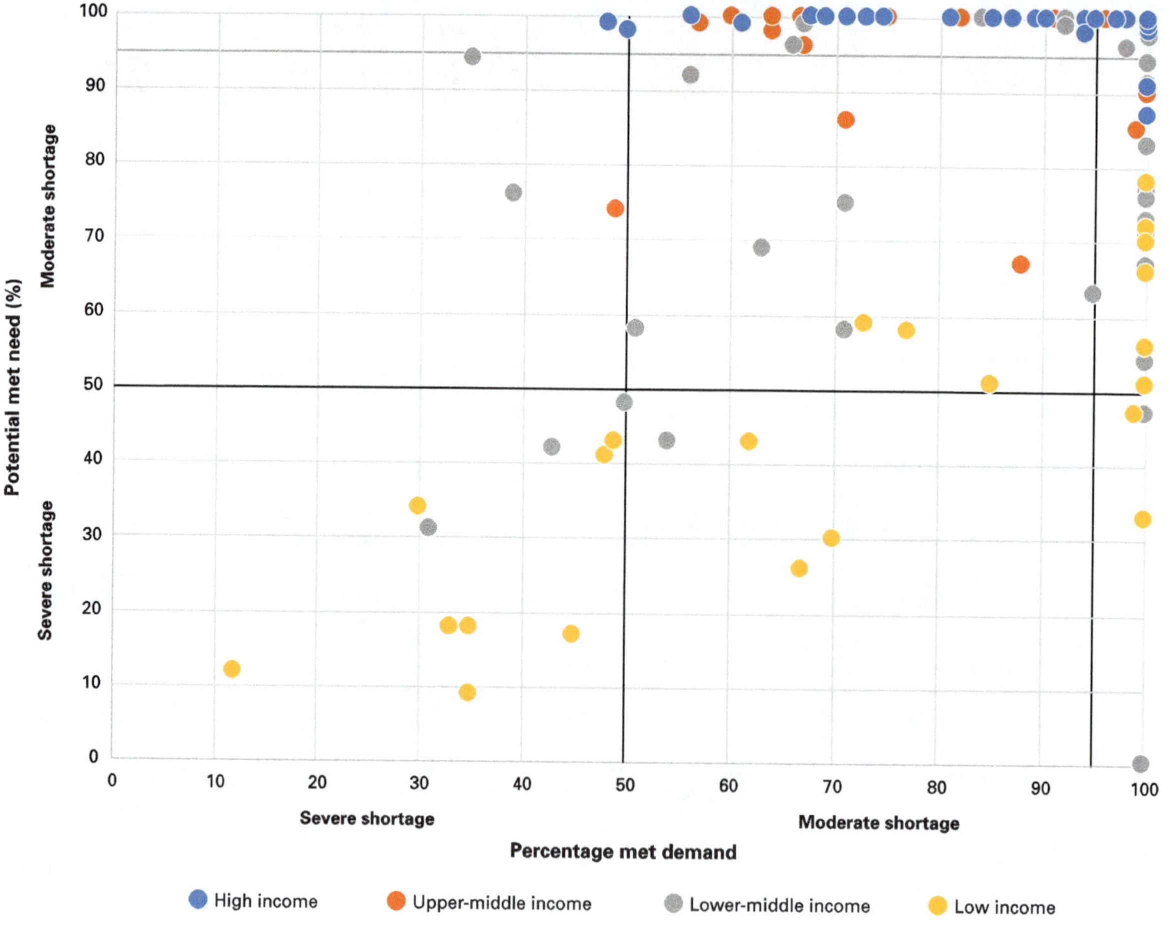

Source: Estimates made for this report.

EQUITY OF ACCESS TO THE SRMNAH WORKFORCE

The SoWMy need and demand calculations presented in Chapter 4 have limitations, not least that they do not take into account within-country inequities in the availability of and access to SRMNAH workers. Unless the workforce is equitably available and accessible to all service users, and able to provide the same quality of care for all, it will not meet all the need for SRMNAH services, regardless of the number of health workers.

From the service user's perspective, the concept of accessibility has several dimensions. Barriers to access can be caused by a lack of: physical accessibility (relating to distance, transport, personal security and other physical challenges); service organization (relating to opening hours, waiting times, referral systems, scopes of practice, confidentiality, stigma etc.); and affordability (relating to user fees, informal payments or other costs associated with seeking care from an SRMNAH worker).

Access or choice can also be limited by provider attitudes and values, for example, towards the service user's personal characteristics (age, sex, sexual orientation, ethnicity, language, disability, gender identity, religion, marital status, HIV status etc.) or their right to access contraception services or comprehensive abortion care (96, 97).

Physical accessibility

Physical accessibility is influenced by political decisions about investment in primary health care and allocation of human resources and infrastructure. Inequitable access can occur for many reasons, including geography, topography, climate, conflict, violence, natural disasters and restricted scopes of practice for primary health-care practitioners.

A notable example of geographic disparities in health workforce availability is that observed between urban and rural areas (98), but even within urban areas there can be inequity due to factors such as poverty and means of transport. Inequitable access directly affects maternal and child health outcomes. For example, it is estimated that only 72% of births to rural women are attended by skilled health personnel, compared with 90% for urban women (5).

> **KEY MESSAGES**
>
> ▸ Workforce data and analyses should be disaggregated by characteristics such as gender, occupation group and geographical location, so that gaps in provision can be identified and addressed.
>
> ▸ Some population groups are at risk of restricted access to SRMNAH workers due to age, poverty, geographical location, disability, ethnicity, conflict, sexual orientation, gender identity, religion etc.
>
> ▸ "Left behind" groups require special attention to ensure that they can access care from qualified practitioners. The SRMNAH workforce requires a supportive policy and working environment, and appropriate education and training, to understand and meet the specific needs of vulnerable groups and thus provide care that is accessible and acceptable to all.
>
> ▸ The voices of service users are essential for understanding the factors that influence their care-seeking behaviour.

National-level estimates can mask geographical and occupational variations: the case of Ghana

Ghana is one of the very few countries that provided workforce data for SoWMy 2021 disaggregated by both occupation group and subnational region. Using these, and subnational estimates for demographic and epidemiologic indicators (101-104), the need for SRMNAH worker time in 2019 was estimated separately for each of Ghana's 10 regions in the same way as for the national estimate, and mapped against availability.

Map A shows that the populous Greater Accra and Ashanti regions had the highest need for SRMNAH worker hours. Map B shows that these two regions also had the most time available from the three main SRMNAH occupation groups combined (midwives, nurses and SRMNAH doctors). Across all occupation groups, the total amount of available time exceeded the amount of time needed, by a considerable margin in five of the regions. However, disaggregation by occupation group showed that this overall positive picture was due mainly to a high supply of nurses. Nurses are of course an important SRMNAH occupation group and can meet some of the need. However, some essential SRMNAH interventions require midwives and doctors, and this analysis highlighted significant needs-based shortages of these occupation groups, with much regional variation.

In contrast to the aggregated figures in Map B, Map C shows that only one region (Upper West) had enough midwives to meet the need, while the Northern region had less than half the midwife time needed. Maps D and E show that the available doctor time was insufficient in all regions: no region had available even half of the needed hours.

Greater Accra and Upper West had the best supplies of general medical practitioners, but even here fewer than half of the needed hours were available. Shortages of obstetricians and gynaecologists were even more serious: again, Greater Accra had the best supply, but only 29% of the needed obstetrician and gynaecologist time was available. The low number of medical practitioners suggests that, if availability were mapped against need at district level, there might be districts without specialists, particularly where there are no hospitals, leaving other health workers to manage obstetric emergencies.

This analysis underlines the importance of disaggregated data as part of health workforce planning, and of monitoring and evaluating efforts to increase equity in health worker availability.

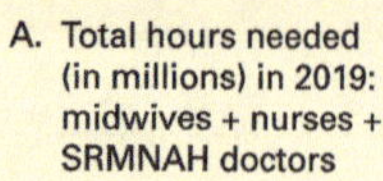

A. Total hours needed (in millions) in 2019: midwives + nurses + SRMNAH doctors

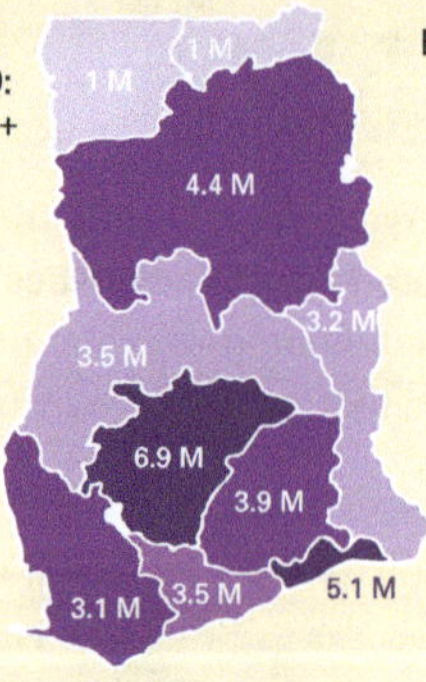

B. Total hours available (in millions) in 2019: midwives + nurses + SRMNAH doctors

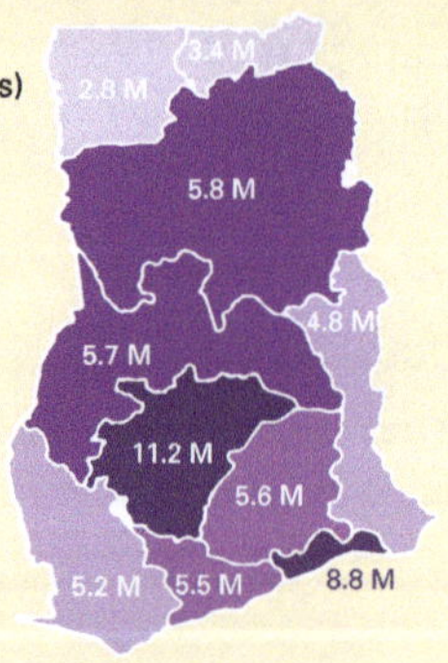

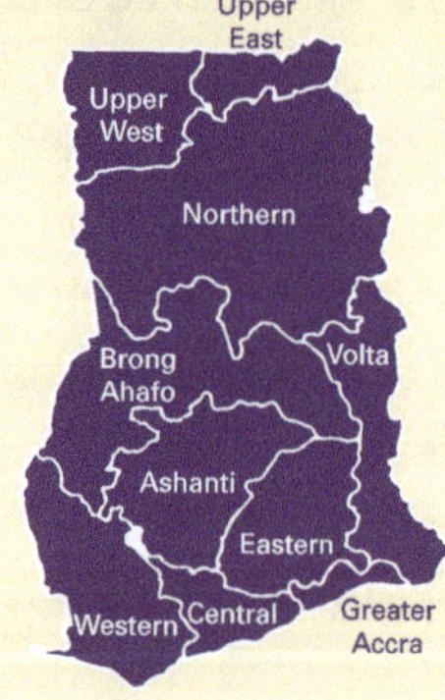

C. Percentage of needed hours which are available: midwives

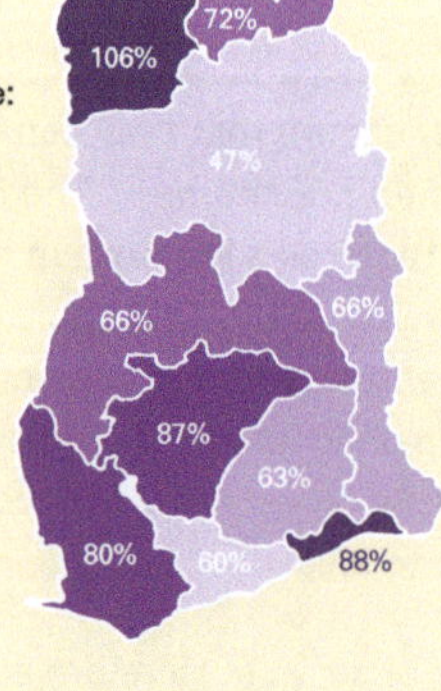

D. Percentage of needed hours which are available: general medical practitioners

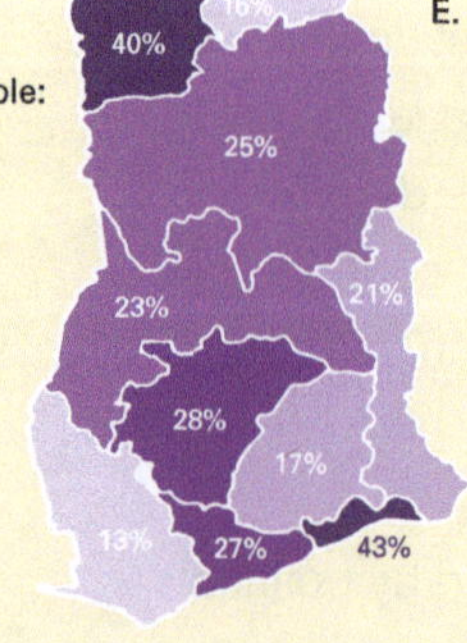

E. Percentage of needed hours which are available: obstetricians and gynaecologists

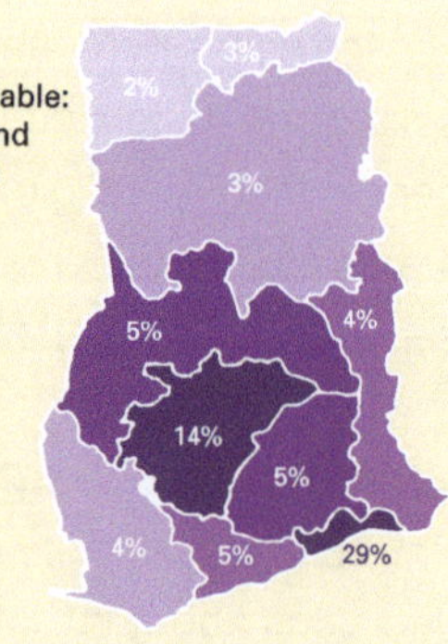

Contributed by Winfred Dotse-Gborgbortsi (WorldPop, School of Geography and Environmental Science, University of Southampton).

With almost half the world's population, and most of the world's poor, living in rural areas, equitable workforce distribution is of paramount importance. WHO has published guidance on increasing accessibility to health workers in remote and rural areas through improved retention *(99)*. A key element of the guidance is rigorous monitoring and evaluation of efforts to increase health worker availability, which requires geographically disaggregated data. Recent advances in the use of geographic information systems to measure and understand geographical variations in access to SRMNAH workers and services provide a significant opportunity *(100)* but investment and commitment are needed to ensure high-quality data and analyses. This is illustrated by the fact that very few countries provided SRMNAH worker data to NHWA that were disaggregated by administrative area. Box 5.1 illustrates the important additional insights made possible by disaggregated data.

Provider attitudes and behaviour

Even if SRMNAH workers are available and accessible, if the care they offer is not acceptable to service users and their communities, then women and adolescents may choose not to use, or may be prevented from using, SRMNAH services. Instead, they may consult unqualified practitioners, or no one at all. Accounts of interactions with SRMNAH workers, whether one's own or other people's, can influence decisions about whether to access services. Such factors are often more influential than distance and cost in decisions about where to give birth and with whom *(105)*, and this can present a significant barrier to access. Some communities have addressed this issue by setting up systems of midwife-led care, by midwives from their own communities, so that service users do not avoid seeking care in systems that discriminate against them *(106, 107)*.

Globally, the percentage of births attended by skilled health personnel has increased *(5)*, but in some settings lack of respectful care discourages women and adolescents from consulting an SRMNAH worker (Box 5.2).

Respectful maternity care

Respectful maternity care is an overarching philosophy, at the core of which is a human-rights based approach to the provision of high-quality, woman- and newborn-centred care *(35, 108)*. The Respectful Maternity Care Charter states that high-quality maternity care supports and upholds the dignity of both the mother and the newborn, and sets out how these human rights should be guaranteed in pregnancy and childbirth care *(109)*. The SRMNAH workforce plays an important role in creating and sustaining care environments that promote respectful maternity care. However, respectful care first requires systems and facilities that respect, not only women and newborns, but also the health workforce: for example, by ensuring effective and safe working environments, freedom from bullying and harassment, supportive supervision and fair compensation.

Health-care settings and interactions can reflect a society's structural gender inequalities, which often mean women, both as health-care users and health workers, have lower social status than men *(110, 111)*. Midwives are often the backbone of maternity services, but when they work in disempowering environments their contributions may not be recognized and rewarded, and they may be unsupported or disrespected by supervisors. Such settings typically offer limited ways to alleviate stress or nurture motivation, which in turn may lead to disrespectful, lower-quality care *(110)*. Moreover, in settings where women experience or fear experiencing mistreatment, they may avoid the health system altogether *(105, 112)*.

During Covid-19, health professionals in many settings have lacked sufficient PPE, and there have been violations of women's rights to respectful maternity care, such as by not allowing labour companions, instituting mandatory separation of the mother and newborn, restricting breastfeeding, and increasing potentially harmful interventions without indication (e.g. caesarean section, instrumental birth, induction and augmentation of labour) *(113)*. Human rights frameworks should guide policy and practice even during a pandemic, to ensure that fundamental rights and best clinical practices are observed in essential maternity services *(114)*. Covid-19 presents an opportunity to critically examine how maternity care services can be transformed to improve quality, equity and the woman-centred nature of care.

Contributed by Meghan A. Bohren (University of Melbourne, Australia) and Özge Tunçalp (WHO).

Midwives' association

The voices of service users are essential for understanding the factors that influence their care-seeking behaviour (Box 5.3).

SRMNAH needs often involve sensitive personal issues, so service users may prefer to consult a health worker of a specific gender. It is therefore important that the SRMNAH workforce includes both men and women, recognizing that an appropriate balance is likely to involve more women than men. In the countries submitting data, 93% of the wider midwifery workforce, 89% of the nursing workforce (excluding those with midwifery training), and 50% of SRMNAH doctors are women. Figure 5.1 shows that this general pattern holds true for all regions and income groups, but there are a few variations. Nurses who are men are most likely to be working in low-income countries. Women SRMNAH doctors are most likely to be working in the African and Western Pacific regions (58% and 55% respectively of SRMNAH doctors are women). In Africa this is mainly due to Algeria and Nigeria, which both report a large number of SRMNAH doctors, of whom two thirds are women. In most other African countries, most SRMNAH doctors are men.

SRMNAH care: global campaign reveals what women want

The global *What Women Want* campaign, led by the White Ribbon Alliance, set out to enquire what women want for their own maternal and reproductive health care, and to demand that their needs are met. Its premise is that women know best about their own health needs and that their knowledge should be heard *(115)*.

The campaign began in India in 2016, where over 100 partners worked together to hear from almost 150,000 women across 24 states. The women generated a long list of demands, 20% of which related to the availability of health workers and 27% to being treated with dignity and respect.

The campaign has since been launched in many more countries, including Kenya, Malawi, Mexico, Nigeria, Pakistan, Uganda and the United Republic of Tanzania. It has so far reached 1.2 million women in 114 countries. It relies on mobilizers from within local communities. The methods they used to listen to women are many and varied: some are conversational and public; others are reflective and private. Every individual woman's ask is recorded, counted and sorted into themes.

A number of the "top 20" themes so far identified are directly relevant to this report. Number 1 is "respectful and dignified care"; number 4 is "increased, competent and better supported midwives and nurses"; number 6 is "increased, competent and better supported doctors" and number 17 is "more female providers". Most of the other themes

relate to the environment in which SRMNAH workers operate. These results clearly show the importance attached by women to the SRMNAH workforce and the quality of the care it is enabled to provide.

In many parts of the world, women are seldom asked about their needs and priorities, so the act of asking the question was affirming for them. Others, however, were tired of being asked but seeing no changes. The campaign calls for policy- and decision-makers at all levels to hear the voices of the participating women and to act on them to drive improvements to health services.

Contributed by Manju Chhugani, Aparajita Gogoi and Kristy Kade (White Ribbon Alliance).

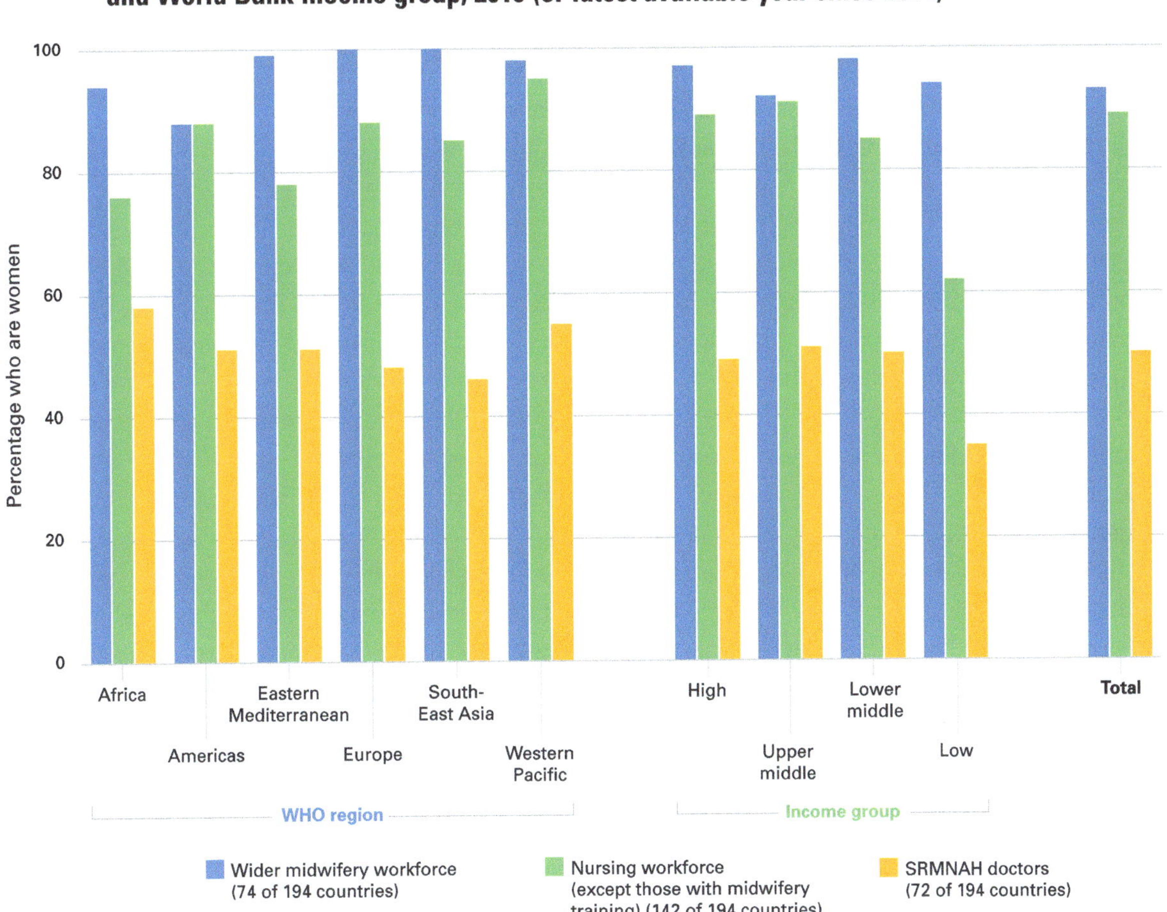

Note: These figures are means, weighted by population size. Thus, large countries have a greater influence on the regional and income group averages than smaller countries.

Source: NHWA, 2020 update.

"Left-behind" groups

Regardless of overall levels of availability and access, vulnerable or marginalized population groups can often be "left behind", resulting in inequities. People can experience discrimination based on a wide range of (often intersecting) characteristics, such as age, gender identity, sexual orientation, race, caste, tribe, ethnicity, religion and disability. Two SoWMy 2021 supplements (https://unfpa.org/sowmy) focus on workforce issues relating to adolescents and to women, newborns and adolescents living in or seeking refuge from humanitarian and fragile settings.

Strategies to address the impact of Covid-19 on access to SRMNAH workers

Continuity of SRMNAH services is critical for women, newborns and adolescents. Even during a global pandemic, women and adolescents need SRMNAH care: service disruption risks eroding hard-fought gains in SRMNAH outcomes (116), potentially leading to an increase in unintended pregnancies, sexually transmitted infections, unsafe abortions and to increased health risks for mothers, newborns and adolescents (117). PMNCH has issued a call to action, urging governments to protect and promote SRMNAH and rights throughout the Covid-19 response and recovery phases (22).

According to a WHO survey (83), by March 2021 94% of 135 responding countries reported some kind of disruption to health services in the preceding 3 months because of Covid-19, and nearly half reported that they had intentionally scaled back provision. Contraceptive services were disrupted in 44% of countries, antenatal services in 39% of countries and facility-based birth services in 25% of countries. The disruptions resulted from a combination of demand and supply factors. On the demand side, 57% of countries reported reductions in outpatient care attendance, but this was less common in 2021 than in an earlier round of data collection in 2020. Other factors mentioned included community fear and mistrust (57% of countries), financial difficulties caused by lockdowns (43%), and supply chain disruptions (29%). Another study estimated that service disruptions due to Covid-19 could result in 2.7 million unsafe abortions *(118)*.

A Global Financing Facility analysis of the impact of Covid-19 on essential health services for women and children drew on data reported by 63,000 health facilities and highlighted similar effects of the pandemic on SRMNAH *(119)*. Their analysis of data to June 2020 showed that the number of women who attended four antenatal care visits during pregnancy dropped in Liberia. In Nigeria, 26% of respondents who needed health services said they could not access the services they needed. Of these, a quarter said this was due to lockdowns and movement restrictions imposed to control the pandemic. Results were mixed across indicators. For example, in Nigeria, contraceptive services decreased by more than

10% in April 2020 and by 15% in May; women giving birth at health facilities decreased by 6%. In Afghanistan, however, while postnatal consultations were not affected by the crisis, outpatient consultations dropped by 14%.

Disruptions to health services and the impact of occupationally acquired infections have taken their toll on health workers *(120, 121)*. A global study of more than 700 maternity care providers in high-, middle- and low-income countries showed the additional challenges posed by the need for knowledge acquisition and communication, especially concerning the care of women, whether or not infected with Covid-19 *(122)*.

The evidence does not yet fully capture the impact of Covid-19 on the health and rights of women, newborns and adolescents. However, because the virus can adversely affect SRMNAH outcomes, it is essential for health authorities to educate SRMNAH workers about the effects of Covid-19 on maternal and newborn health care *(123)* and on their own physical and mental health while working in this new environment. WHO has issued interim guidance on using routine data to monitor the effects of Covid-19 on essential health services, including SRMNAH *(124)*.

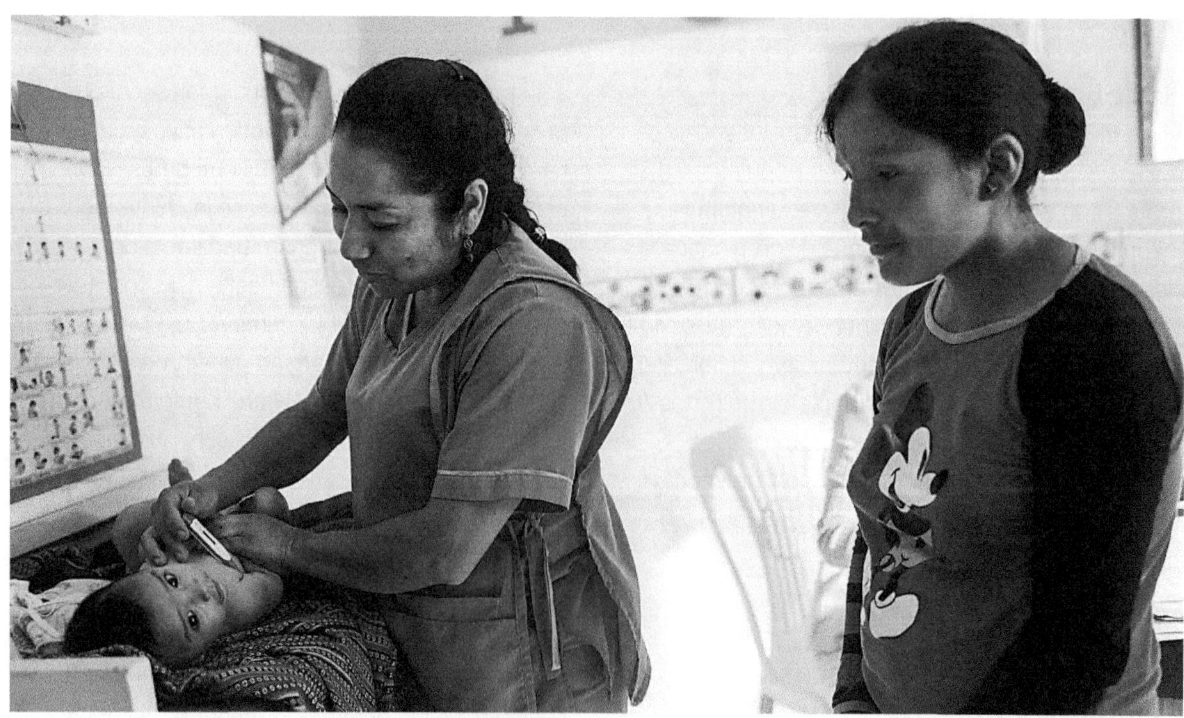

Health check at a clinic in Potracancha, Huanuco Region, Peru.
© Gates Archive/Mark Makela.

ENABLING AND EMPOWERING THE SRMNAH WORKFORCE: GENDER MATTERS

The health workforce is on average 70% women, although there are gender differences by occupation *(125)*. Women account for 93% of midwives and 89% of nurses, compared with 50% of SRMNAH doctors (see Chapter 5). The considerable gendered disparities in pay rates, career pathways and decision-making power create systemic inefficiencies by limiting the productivity, distribution, motivation and retention of female health workers *(126)*.

Investment in the health workforce can boost inclusive economic growth, mainly due to job creation, particularly for women and young people *(17, 127)*. Increasing the education and employment of midwives will play an important role in ensuring gender equality in pay and position. However, the persistent gender biases and the lack of recognition and undervaluing of women's unpaid and informal work need to be acknowledged and addressed. Significant social, cultural, economic and professional barriers, including gender inequality, are known to prevent the provision of high-quality midwifery care in low- and middle-income countries *(57)*. This chapter provides an overview of the key issues involved in enabling and empowering the midwifery workforce by gender-transformative policies and other measures.

Recent analyses have highlighted several critical issues for midwives: leadership; decent work, free from all forms of discrimination and harassment, including sexual harassment; gender pay gaps; and occupational segregation across the entire workforce, which has specific resonance for SRMNAH *(128, 129)*. Gender-transformative

health workforce policies and measures must be implemented in order to reach global UHC targets, especially for women and newborns.

The Covid-19 pandemic has also had a disproportionate impact on women, especially in terms of employment security, increased caring and home-schooling responsibilities, and increased incidences of gender-based

> ### ⌕ KEY MESSAGES
>
> ▶ The health workforce is on average 70% women, with gender differences by occupation. Midwives are more likely to be women; they experience considerable gendered disparities in pay rates, career pathways and decision-making power.
>
> ▶ Only half of reporting countries have midwife leaders within the national Ministry of Health. Limited opportunities for midwives to hold leadership positions and the scarcity of women who are role models in leadership positions hinder midwives' career advancement and their ability to work to their full potential.
>
> ▶ Access to decent work that is free from violence and discrimination is essential to address gender-related barriers and challenges. All countries need policies to prevent attacks on health workers.
>
> ▶ A gender transformative policy environment will challenge the underlying causes of gender inequities, guarantee the human rights, agency and well-being of caregivers, both paid and unpaid, recognize the value of health work and of women's work, and reward adequately.

Midwives' association

violence, especially in the home. In addition, the pandemic has affected the health of health-care workers, especially women. Unsafe working conditions reported include lack of access to effective personal protective equipment, long hours, isolation from family and violence and harassment towards health workers *(130)*. It is likely that such conditions have led to women leaving the profession or moving into non-clinical roles *(131, 132)*.

Occupational segregation by gender

Occupational segregation by gender is driven by long-standing gender norms that define caring as women's work and portraying men as more suited to technical specialties, such as medicine *(128)*. Midwifery, and the role of caring for women and newborns, is often undervalued, leading to midwives having no voice and no place at the leadership table: this hinders respect, access to decent work and pay equity.

The majority of physicians, dentists and pharmacists are men, whereas nearly all midwives and most nurses are women *(125)*. Health occupation groups consisting predominantly of women are assigned lower social value, power and pay than those consisting predominantly of men. Women health workers often have multiple roles: being chief caregivers for children, needing and wanting to be economically productive while also managing community expectations that they will do unpaid work. Midwifery in particular is seen as "women's work" *(133, 134)* which often confuses and undervalues midwives' economic and professional contributions to society *(57)*.

Gender segregation often results in restriction of choices and job opportunities for midwives and reinforces unequal power structures within society *(128)*. Gendered workplace hierarchies *(135)* and social, economic and professional barriers often prevent midwives from working to their full potential, and cause frustration in the workplace, leading to either attrition or further embedding of stereotypes. Midwives can lack professional autonomy within the health workforce if their capacities and skills are unrecognized or undervalued by medical and other institutional hierarchies *(129)*. Professional autonomy is established in national regulations, such as those on scope of practice, but these regulations may be influenced by medical or other institutional hierarchies. The voices of midwives make it clear that "power, agency and status" are vitally important for midwives if progress is to be made in delivering high-quality care *(129)*.

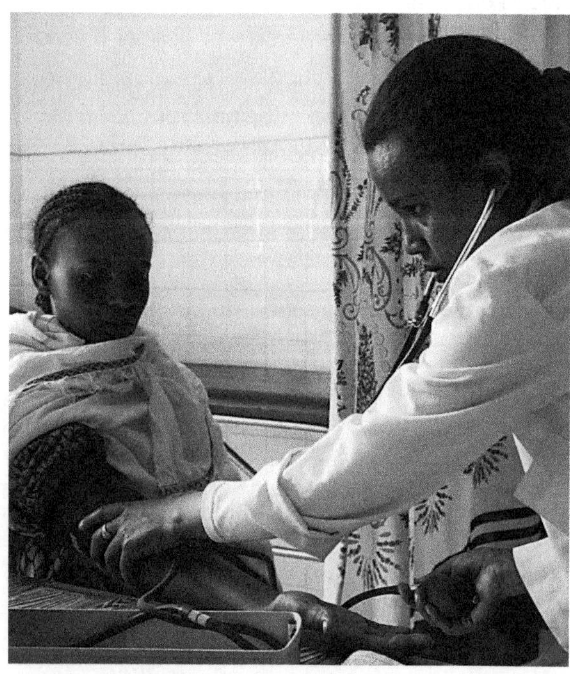

Midwife performing an antenatal check at a clinic in Gebre Guracha village, Oromia Region, Ethiopia.
© Bill & Melinda Gates Foundation/Prashant Panjiar.

Midwife leadership

Health-care leadership is essential to enable midwives to work to their full potential. While 70% of the health and social care workforce are women, just 25% of senior roles are held by women *(128)*. The number of countries with midwives in leadership roles (see glossary) was explored in the ICM member association survey. Of the 80 countries providing data, most (71%) reported at least one midwife leader at some level (in the national Ministry of Health, subnational health ministry offices, regulatory authority or health facilities). Most of the remainder (20%) could not obtain this information, leaving 9% reporting no midwives in leadership positions at any level. Table 6.1 shows that countries were most likely to have midwives in leadership positions at the health facility level; just over half had midwife leaders in the Ministry of Health or regulatory authorities. Midwife leaders were most likely to be reported by countries in the Americas and Eastern Mediterranean regions, but small numbers of reporting countries mean that these results may not be representative of all countries in these regions. Appointing senior midwives as leaders at country level would provide a significant lever for building capacity.

Limited opportunities for leadership and the scarcity of women leaders as role models hinder midwives' ability to climb the leadership ladder. It is also likely that when no midwives hold mid-level leadership positions, such as at the district/provincial level, there is a significant gap in the ability of these levels to provide supportive supervision and mentoring to midwives and the ability to make good decisions on issues that affect midwives.

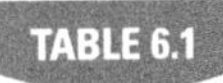

Percentage of 80 countries with midwives in leadership positions, by WHO region and World Bank income group, 2019–2020

	Number of countries reporting/total	% of countries with midwives in leadership in...				
		National MoH	Subnational MoH	Regulatory authority	Health facilities	Any level
WHO REGION						
Africa	29/47	66%	52%	45%	62%	69%
Americas	12/35	75%	75%	67%	92%	92%
Eastern Mediterranean	8/21	50%	75%	63%	63%	88%
Europe	13/53	15%	23%	54%	46%	54%
South-East Asia	7/11	29%	71%	43%	71%	57%
Western Pacific	11/27	45%	64%	64%	73%	73%
INCOME GROUP						
High	19/61	21%	42%	68%	58%	63%
Upper middle	12/55	75%	75%	67%	75%	83%
Lower middle	29/49	48%	52%	45%	55%	66%
Low	20/29	70%	65%	45%	60%	80%
TOTAL	**80/194**	**51%**	**56%**	**54%**	**60%**	**71%**

MoH = Ministry of Health.

Note: A few countries reported "don't know": they are included in the denominators for the above percentages. They may have midwife leaders, but were unable to specify how many.

Source: ICM survey.

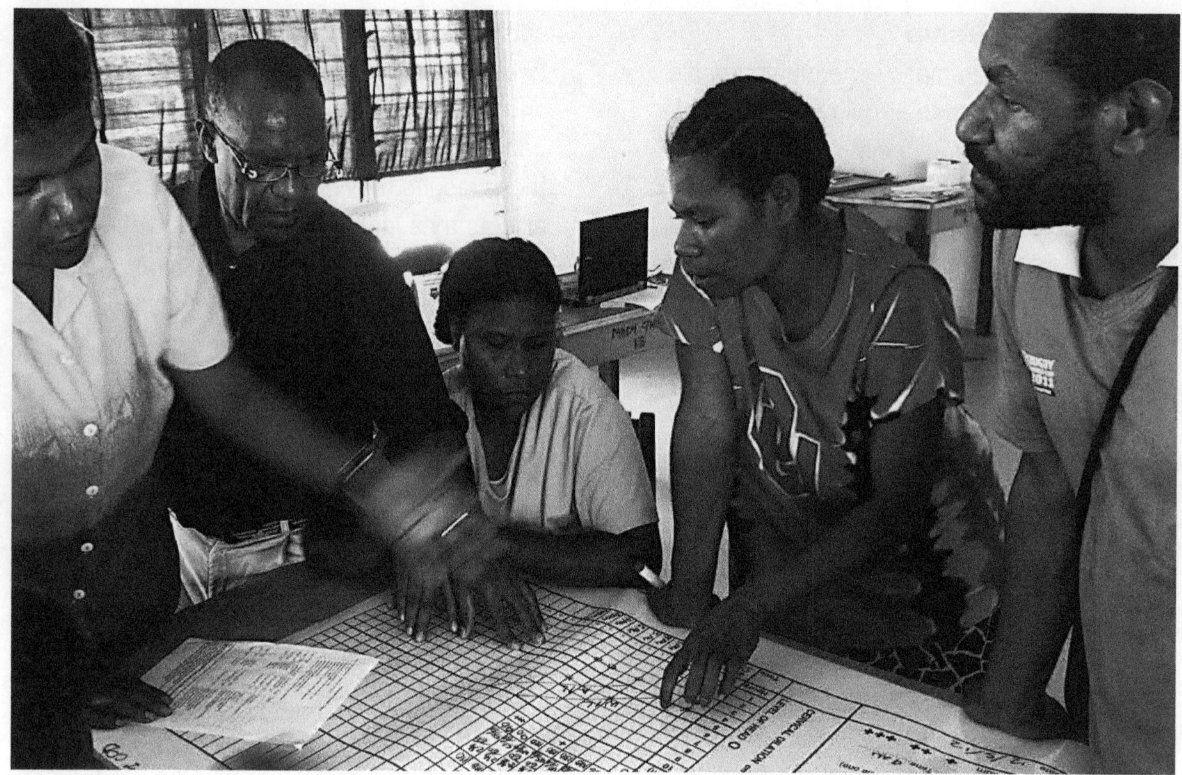

Training of SRMNAH workers in Papua New Guinea.
© Heather Gulliver.

The intersection of issues such as gender, ethnicity, age, geographic location and socioeconomic status contributes to multiple layers of disadvantage, including aspects of occupational segregation. Women are more likely to work part-time: an additional barrier to accessing formal leadership roles *(125)*. Lack of investment in women's professional development, especially in developing and utilizing leadership skills, inhibits them from advocating their case *(136)* and further perpetuates gender segregation. Some midwives have expressed concern that leadership opportunities can be limited in countries where midwifery is subsumed within nursing structures *(129)*.

The ICM Young Midwife Leaders programme is an example of support for midwives in developing their leadership skills (Box 6.1).

Decent work

Decent working conditions in the health sector are fundamental for providing high-quality and effective care. Decent work deficits are among the key reasons why almost all countries face challenges in recruiting, deploying and retaining enough well trained and motivated health workers *(137)*.

The ability to access decent work, free from violence and discrimination, is essential in order to address gender-related barriers and challenges for the SRMNAH workforce *(128)*. Violence in the workplace affects all health workers but is particularly harmful to women *(136)*. Sexual harassment in the workplace also causes harm, ill health, attrition, low morale and stress. Gender power relations and their intersectionality with other factors, such as age, marital status, ethnicity and income, although often invisible, have been shown to be associated with the type and source of violence experienced by women working in health professions *(136, 138)*. In 2019, the International Labour Conference adopted a new convention and recommendation to combat violence and harassment in the workplace. It is the first international treaty to proclaim the right to work free from violence and harassment, including gender-based violence and harassment. The health sector is recognized as involving a high risk of exposure to violence and harassment: the treaty calls on members to adopt measures to combat that risk *(139)*.

Building the next generation of midwife leaders

ICM's Young Midwife Leaders (YML) programme enables young midwives (aged under 35) from low- and middle-income countries to learn how to develop as leaders of the profession and to strengthen their national midwives' associations. The objectives of the ICM programme are to:

- increase leadership-related knowledge, skills and self-confidence (e.g. for strategic planning, project management and policy advocacy);
- increase awareness of health systems; and
- increase commitment to the professionalism of midwives, their education, the policies that govern them, national/regional midwives' associations and the health system in which they operate.

In addition to the global programme led by ICM, UNFPA supports a YML programme in 11 countries in Latin America and the Caribbean and six states in Mexico. Several cohorts have now benefited from the programme. It is anticipated that the alumni will form a global community of young midwife advocates, sharing ideas and experiences to transform midwifery. Below, some young midwives share their views of the YML programme.

Sandra Blanco
MEXICO
"It was a great opportunity to develop my skills in mentoring, follow-up, leadership and management."

Sylvia Hamata
NAMIBIA
"Being a YML has enhanced my emotional intelligence and self-confidence to use my voice and skills to advocate without fear for the midwifery workforce and for women and newborns. Being exposed and linked to the global community has widened my knowledge of the impact of midwives' work on maternal and newborn well-being."

Bartholomew Kamlewe
ZAMBIA
"Exposure to online leadership courses and webinars has led to a marked increase in my knowledge about midwifery issues from a global perspective and increased my advocacy skills for maternal and newborn issues."

Sandra Lopez
PARAGUAY
"The main objective of the programme was to raise the visibility of midwives, so that society recognizes their existence, importance and functions."

Andrea Mateos Orbegoso
PERU
"The YML programme motivated both my personal and my professional life. Meeting young midwives from other countries in the region who were just starting their careers helped me understand the needs of the profession and how I could contribute."

Tekla Shiindi-Mbidi
NAMIBIA
"The YML programme has presented me with an amazing opportunity. My perspective about midwifery has completely changed and I am now able to speak confidently for and about midwives, the midwifery profession and practice. I have grown a global network of both young and experienced midwives, including global leaders in midwifery."

Luseshelo Simwinga
MALAWI
"The YML programme empowered me to become a proactive midwifery leader, to advocate for the rights of childbearing women and newborns and for dignified care. The programme has also provided me with perfect networks which I can tap into to gain midwifery knowledge for my everyday practice."

Samson Udho
UGANDA
"The YML programme has transformed my networking and leadership abilities. I feel more grounded as a leader, and able to transform ideas into practical and sustainable actions that strengthen my career as well as the midwifery profession."

Contributed by Ann Yates (ICM), Alma Virginia Camacho-Hübner (UNFPA) and Joyce Thompson (UNFPA consultant).

Despite this international focus on violence and harassment in the workplace, only half (52%) of 164 countries providing data in NHWA have national or subnational policies to prevent attacks on health workers, with a further 10% saying this is partially true. Figure 6.1 shows that countries in South-East Asia and the Eastern Mediterranean are most likely to have these measures in place and that they are most common in high-income countries (65%, compared with 47% of low- and middle-income countries).

Gender inequalities increase the risk of an unsafe work environment due to some of the issues noted above, including lack of opportunity and recognition, low or unequal pay, precarious work environments and lack of job security *(136)*. As noted in previous chapters, there is a lack of data on the SRMNAH workforce, and the data that do exist are rarely disaggregated by gender and profession.

The trade union movement is an important force for negotiating decent conditions. Many countries lack laws requiring and promoting gender equality at work. Health workers who are men are more likely than those who are women to be organized in trade unions and therefore more likely to advocate for pay and conditions that suit men *(128)*. The absence of collective bargaining in many countries leads to gender pay gaps that put women at a lifelong economic disadvantage.

Social dialogue is key to achieving decent working conditions. The main goal of social dialogue is to promote consensus building and democratic involvement among the main stakeholders in the world of work. Box 6.2 provides examples of how social dialogue has been applied for midwives.

Ensuring that midwives, as well as their employers and other relevant stakeholders, have an opportunity to make their voices heard is critical for enabling them to play a full and active role in shaping and developing the SRMNAH workforce. The 1977 Nursing Personnel Convention *(145)*, where applicable to the SRMNAH workforce, calls for the promotion of personnel participation in the

---

Figure 6.1 **Existence of national or subnational policies or laws in 164 countries for the prevention of attacks on health workers, 2019, by WHO region and World Bank income group**

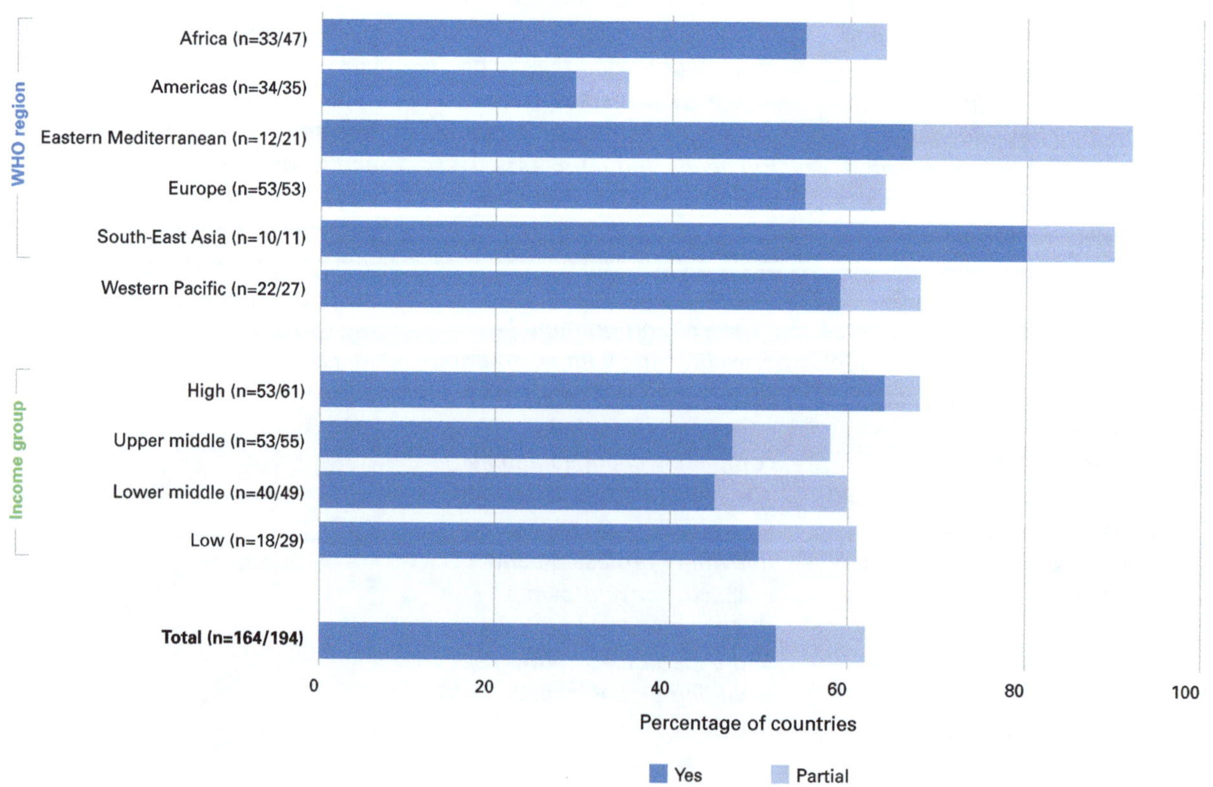

Source: NHWA, 2020 update.

planning of broader health and nursing policies. It provides for negotiation as a means to determine working conditions and establishes dispute settlement mechanisms. Midwives who are also nurses are covered by this convention; future work is to be undertaken to include midwives explicitly in these provisions.

Gender pay gap

The gender pay gap is not unique to health care, but reports suggest that the gap is larger in health care than in other sectors *(125, 128)*. The gender pay gap is driven by women being employed in lower-status or lower-paid roles, further highlighting the intersection with occupational segregation. Box 6.3 highlights these pay inequities in Morocco and Tunisia. Unpaid health and social care also contributes to the gender pay gap in health and care work *(146)*.

Midwives have reported earnings that are lower than those in similar professions, sometimes requiring them to depend on other sources of income to survive, or to charge informal payments. Such situations can add to the pressure and exhaustion experienced by midwives and reduce their accessibility to women, newborns and adolescents. In low- and middle-income countries, midwives have reported not being reimbursed through government insurance programmes. Those midwives either prioritized caring for women who could pay them directly or took on loans, risking personal financial stress *(129)*.

These issues are not unique to low- and middle-income countries. Midwives in some high-income countries have complained publicly about inequitable pay and sought to address the structural barriers that contribute to pay inequity *(147, 148)*. In New Zealand this issue reached the country's High Court: agreement was reached committing the parties to co-design a new model following pay equity principles, and discussions are ongoing.

Towards gender transformative policies

Most of the gender biases and gaps referred to in this chapter reflect an inequitable system and have persisted for decades. They call for a reformed system and work environment that creates decent working conditions for women and closes gender gaps in leadership and pay *(128)*. A gender transformative policy environment is needed that will challenge the underlying causes of gender inequities, guarantee the human rights, agency and well-being of caregivers, both paid and unpaid, recognize the real value of health work and of women's work, and reward adequately *(128, 146, 149)*.

BOX 6.2

The importance of social dialogue

Social dialogue can positively contribute to the development and reform of health services. Social dialogue brings governments, employers' and workers' organizations and other policy leaders together to reach agreements about matters on which they have different views *(140)*. The freedom of health workers to express their concerns and to organize and participate freely in social dialogue are guaranteed in the fundamental rights to freedom of association and the effective recognition of the right to collective bargaining *(141)*.

Effective social dialogue requires strong, representative and independent social partners *(137)*.

Around the world, workers' organizations are actively engaging in social dialogue with employers' organizations and governments. In 2018, the Midwifery Employee Representation and Advisory Service (a union representing midwives in New Zealand) signed a multiemployer collective agreement with district health boards. The three-year agreement covers topics concerning safe staffing, hours of work, including breaks and rest periods, salary and allowances, leave, and education, training and development. It aims to ensure sustainable and responsible workforce development to provide high-quality health care *(142)*. The Malta Union of Midwives and Nurses signed a five-year sectoral agreement with the Ministry of Health in 2018 that aims to substantially improve working conditions for nurses and midwives working within public services *(143)*. Within the German United Services Trade Union, regional interest groups specifically for midwives were established to strengthen the visibility and voice of midwives within the union *(144)*.

Salary variations between SRMNAH professionals: the cases of Morocco and Tunisia

Comparing the salaries of different SRMNAH professionals in two middle-income countries that have relatively well developed health workforces (Morocco and Tunisia) highlights inequalities. The table below shows the gross monthly starting salary for public sector workers, comparing midwives, general practitioners and obstetricians and gynaecologists. It also compares these salaries to the *Salaire Minimum Interprofessionnel Garanti* (SMIG), the minimum guaranteed public sector salary, which is enshrined in law.

	Morocco		Tunisia		Salary compared to SMIG	
	Moroccan dirhams	US dollar equivalent	Tunisian dinars	US dollar equivalent	Morocco	Tunisia
SMIG	2517.00	283.47	348.00	128.76	-	-
Midwife	6129.32	686.32	1800.00	664.74	x 2.42	x 5.16
General practitioner	8786.78	983.89	3454.00	1275.56	x 3.47	x 9.90
Obstetrician and gynaecologist	14915.00	1670.09	4055.00	1487.51	x 5.89	x 11.55

SMIG = public sector minimum wage.

Note: Salary data were provided via personal communication in 2021 with UNFPA Morocco, UNFPA Tunisia and the Tunisian Ministry of Health.

Midwives earn just over double the SMIG in Morocco, but five times the SMIG in Tunisia. For general practitioners, the salary is 3.5 times the SMIG in Morocco but almost 10 times in Tunisia. Obstetricians and gynaecologists earn around six times the SMIG in Morocco but more than 11 times the SMIG in Tunisia.

Contributed by Atf Ghérissi (independent consultant) and Mohamed Afifi (UNFPA Arab States Regional Office).

Good-quality employment that promotes gender equality and benefits all parties (service users, care workers and unpaid carers) is both possible and feasible *(146)*. The International Labour Organization has developed the 5R Framework for Decent Care Work, which calls for such a transformative policy environment by: recognizing, reducing and redistributing unpaid care work; rewarding paid care work; promoting more and decent work for care workers; and guaranteeing care workers' representation, social dialogue and collective bargaining *(146)*. A career pathway for midwives needs to be developed in every country, providing opportunities for growth and development, and to provide visible and effective role models for midwives and other young women. This would allow them to play a major transformative role in the profession and thereby contribute to gender equity in the workforce.

Some of these transformative policies and examples have direct relevance for the SRMNAH workforce. These include: social protection transfers and subsidies for workers with family responsibilities; labour regulations, including leave policies and other family-friendly working arrangements enabling a better balance between work and family lives; the strengthening of collective bargaining in care sectors; and the building of alliances between trade unions representing care workers and civil society organizations representing care recipients and unpaid carers. Directly relevant to the needs of midwives are: policy direction that negotiates and implements decent terms and conditions of employment and achieves equal pay for work of equal value for all SRMNAH workers; and ensuring a safe, attractive and stimulating work environment for all. Enabling full and effective participation and equal opportunities for leadership at all levels of decision-making in political, economic and public life is critical and highly relevant. Midwives must be at every table where decisions relating to SRMNAH and maternity services are made.

Progress since 2011

SoWMy 2021 is the third in the SoWMy series of reports. The first (SoWMy 2011) called for investments in midwifery education and regulation and in midwives' associations, especially to improve quality of care. There has been some progress here, with greater recognition of the importance of quality in addition to quantity. In SoWMy 2021, 79% of countries report having a master list of accredited health worker education institutions (although these are not specific to midwifery). SoWMy 2011 called for the recognition of midwifery as a distinct profession, with posts at the national policy level. SoWMy 2021 reports that most countries recognize midwifery as being distinct from nursing, and half have midwives in leadership positions at national level.

On the other hand, there is still a lack of action towards critical areas recommended in 2011, including: costing midwifery and midwives in national health plans; ensuring adequate availability and distribution of suitably equipped health facilities; and improving workforce data. Similarly, 2011 recommendations included: ensuring that midwifery graduates are proficient in all the essential competencies required by their government and regulatory body; using globally recognized standards to improve quality and capacity, with attention to theory–practice balance; recruiting teachers, trainers and tutors, and maintaining and upgrading their competencies in midwifery and transformative education; promoting research and academic activities; and supporting the development of midwifery leadership. Disappointingly, of 75

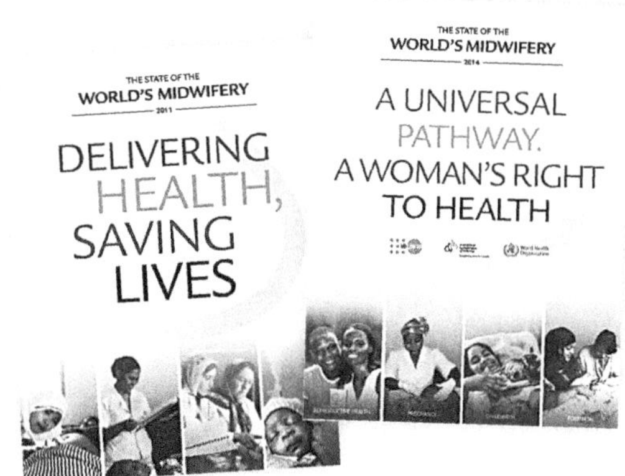

reporting countries, only 24 have a system requiring regular relicensing for midwives with proof of continuing professional development, highlighting the necessity for these issues to reappear in the 2021 recommendations.

Strengthening and enabling midwives' associations to provide much needed leadership, partnership with women and advocacy has been a strong theme in SoWMy. The 2011 report highlighted that associations could raise midwives' profile and status in the national policy arena and strengthen their input into health plans and policy development. Midwives' associations are essential for effective collaboration with other professional associations, with regional and international federations, and with women and communities. SoWMy 2011 also emphasized the need to establish solid governance of midwives' associations, strengthening their administrative capacity and improving financial management. These issues remain current and relevant.

In 2014, SoWMy reported that few low- and middle-income countries had enough SRMNAH workers to meet the need: this remains true in 2021. Many countries show improved workforce availability since 2014, but others have stagnated

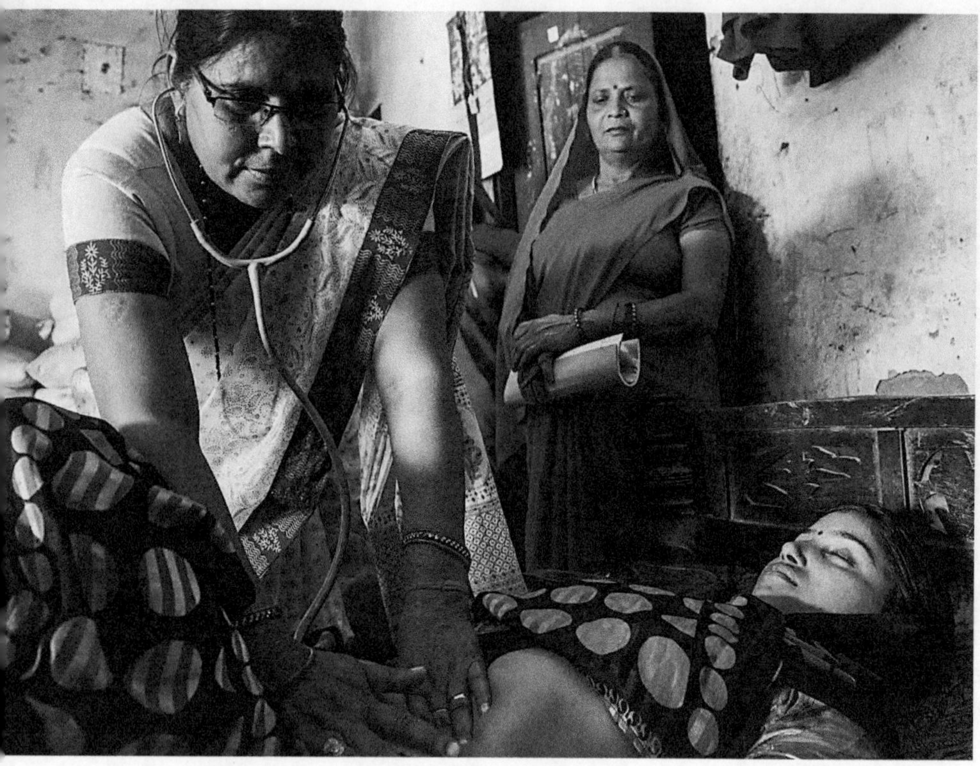

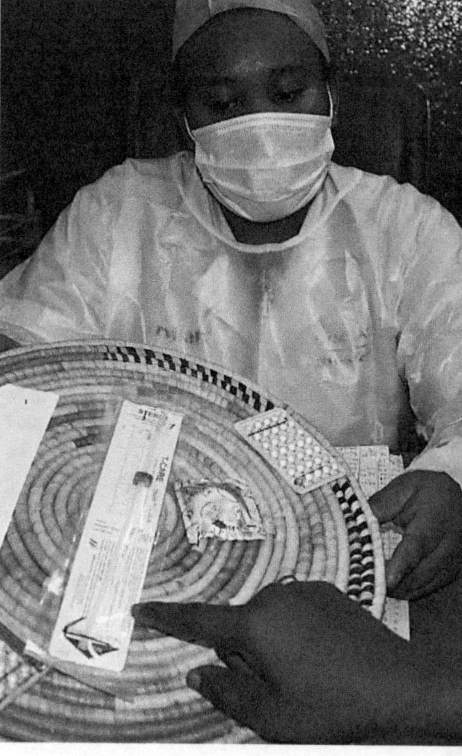

Auxiliary nurse-midwife Archana Verma during an antenatal care visit to the client Babli's home in Kamrawan village, Barabanki District, Uttar Pradesh, India. © Bill & Melinda Gates Foundation/Prashant Panjiar.

Explaining contraceptive options at Ratoma Hospital, Conakry, Guinea. © UNFPA Guinea.

and some show worse availability because workforce growth is not keeping pace with population growth. SoWMy 2014 called for comprehensive, disaggregated data, with the articulation of 10 essential data items to be reported by every country. This has not occurred and the urgent need for improved data remains a key issue in 2021.

SoWMy 2014 showed that midwifery was a "best buy" in primary health care; the evidence presented in SoWMy 2021 strengthens this message. It shows that investing in midwives contributes to achieving a "grand convergence": ending preventable maternal and newborn deaths and improving health and well-being.

SoWMy 2014 introduced the *Midwifery2030* pathway (reproduced on the inside back cover of this report), starting from the premise that pregnant women are healthy unless complications arise and therefore require preventive and supportive care with access to emergency care when needed. Midwifery promotes woman-centred and midwife-led models of care, which achieve excellent outcomes at a lower cost than medicalized models. The pathway remains valid in

2021. The recommendations in this report all aim to make *Midwifery2030* a reality for all countries.

SoWMy 2021 shows that, if available in sufficient numbers, and if educated and regulated according to recognized standards and working across their whole scope of practice as part of an integrated team within an enabling environment, midwives could meet about 90% of the global need for essential SRMNAH interventions (see Webappendices 3 and 5). Despite this massive potential, Chapter 4 shows that midwives comprise a small minority of the global SRMNAH workforce. The "potential met need" estimates reported in Chapter 4 and the country profiles assume that SRMNAH workers have high-quality education and regulatory systems and work within a supportive and enabling environment, but this is not always the case for midwives. Concerted action in each of these key domains is needed in many countries to increase the supply of and demand for midwives and to ensure that they can work to their full potential. Only then will health systems enjoy the full benefit of the uniquely valuable contribution that midwives can make.

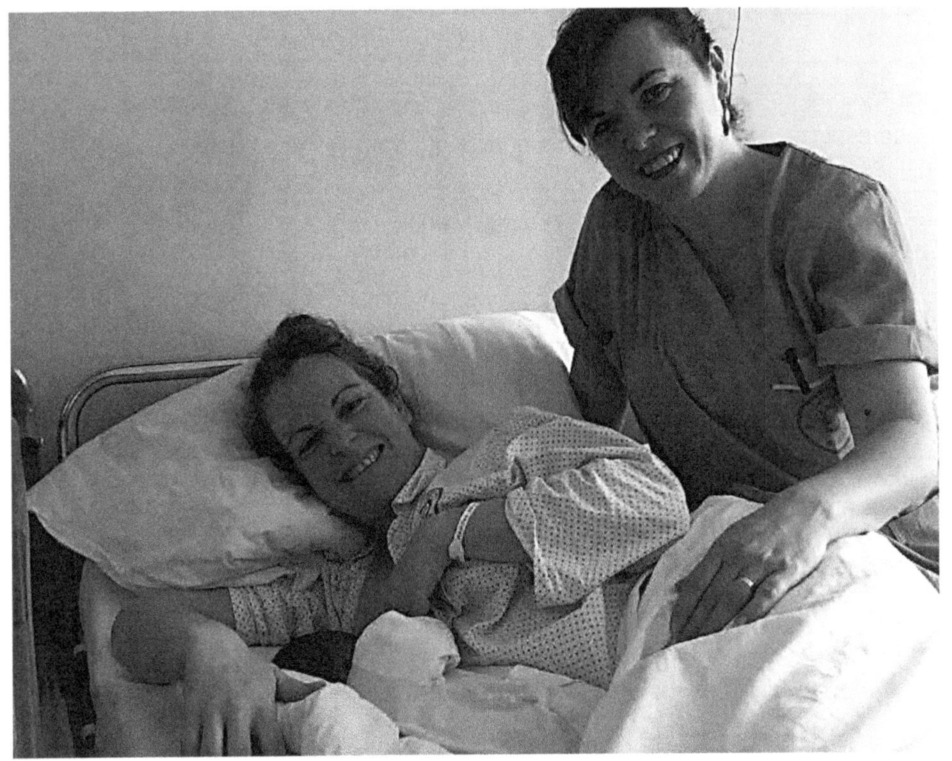

Early initiation of breastfeeding, Croatia. © Natasha Objava.

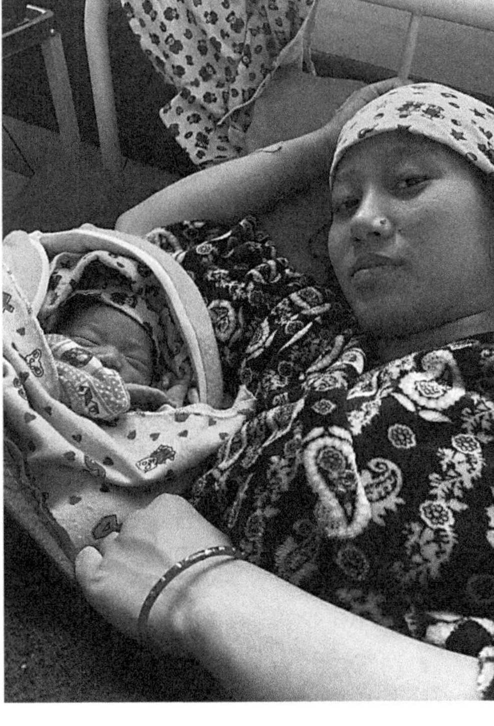

Mother and newborn in Kathmandu, Nepal.
© Felicity Copeland.

This is the first SoWMy report to which all WHO Member States were invited to participate. Low-, middle- and high-income countries show differences, especially in access to resources, workforce shortages, met need and health outcomes. However, there are also many similarities, including the ongoing need to focus on education, regulation and leadership. Constraints to making full use of the SRMNAH workforce vary by country income group; restrictions to midwives' scope of practice can negatively affect both their autonomy and models of care.

Gender imbalances in the SRMNAH workforce (as in the wider health workforce) highlight the need for a gender transformative policy environment, especially for midwives, who are nearly all women. This report also draws attention to the importance of decent work that is free from violence and discrimination, and the need to utilize social dialogue as a means to promote consensus building and democratic involvement and to empower the workforce.

Building back better from the impact of Covid-19

When the Covid-19 pandemic has been brought under control and the world begins to build resilience to future health shocks, there will be a unique opportunity to rebuild and transform SRMNAH services. As part of this effort, investment in growing and optimizing the SRMNAH workforce will be essential.

Covid-19 has shone a light on the importance of investing in primary health care for meeting population health needs. Midwives are essential providers of primary health care and can play a major role in advancing it, especially if enabled to contribute to meeting a broad range of SRMNAH needs in addition to maternity care.

This report describes how the pandemic has led to new ways of delivering SRMNAH services and providing midwife education and training. Robust evaluation of the advantages and disadvantages of these innovations, and retention of those shown to be beneficial, may help to improve the quality and accessibility of services and education programmes.

Bold investments are needed as we look forward to 2030

SoWMy 2021 calls for a strong focus on universal access to essential SRMNAH services, addressing equity at all levels, and leaving no one behind. The evidence in this report can be used to support national and subnational efforts to strengthen the SRMNAH workforce, especially midwives.

To address the global midwife shortage and improve accessibility and quality of care, greater investment in midwives is needed in four key areas: education and training; planning, management and regulation

Four areas of greater investment:

INVEST IN

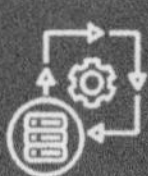

Health workforce planning, management and regulation and in the work environment

INVEST IN

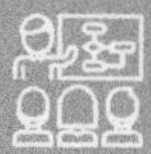

High-quality education and training of midwives

Health workforce data systems

- Collect a minimum health workforce data set which permits disaggregation by occupation group and location, including the following data items: density; graduation rate from education and training programmes; graduates starting practice within one year; duration of education and training; entry rate for foreign health workers; and voluntary and involuntary exit rates from the health labour market.

- Strengthen health workforce data systems and distinguish clearly between midwives and nurses, and nurse-midwives where applicable, to inform decisions about the appropriate skill mix and distribution of health workers to meet population health needs. A specific ISCO code for nurse-midwives could help with this.

- Capture and analyse the various non-clinical roles of midwives, such as in education, management, policy, research, regulation, midwives' associations and government; all these roles are important for the development of the profession.

- Improve understanding of the amount of time devoted by different occupation groups to SRMNAH.

Health workforce planning approaches that reflect the autonomy and professional scope of midwives

- Develop midwife deployment plans that leverage the autonomy of midwives and the wide scope of SRMNAH services they can provide.

- Ensure collaboration between education providers and health workforce planners at the relevant levels of the health system, to secure alignment between graduate numbers and capacity to employ them.

Primary health care, especially in underserved areas

- Organize teams so that midwives can provide the majority of SRMNAH interventions, with access to consultation and referral mechanisms when needed. In many countries, this will include basic emergency obstetric and newborn care services at the primary health-care level.

- Deploy midwives and other SRMNAH specialists such as sexual health nurses and neonatal nurses close to where women and adolescents live.

- Develop and implement strategies to recruit and retain midwives in locations where they are most needed.

Enabling and gender-transformative work environments

- Develop a gender-transformative policy environment to challenge the underlying causes of gender inequality in the health workforce.

- Create career pathways for midwives and link these to educational opportunities and career advancement.

Effective regulatory systems

- Protect the public with regulation that reserves the title "midwife" for those who meet established standards and supports midwives in working to their full scope of practice.

- Use regulatory processes to ensure continuing competence and continuing professional development for midwives.

Educators and trainers

- Ensure that all midwife educators and trainers are equipped with the skills and knowledge they need for teaching and are able to maintain their own professional competencies.

- Create career paths that encourage and facilitate midwives to become educators and trainers of the next generation of midwives.

- Ensure that there are sufficient experienced and skilled preceptors to provide guidance and supervision during clinical placements.

Education and training institutions

- Create and/or strengthen accreditation mechanisms for both public and private sector education and training providers, to ensure that midwives meet established standards for competence and can confidently provide high-quality care to the full extent of their scope of practice.

- Design curricula to include: interdisciplinary modules to build collaboration, increase understanding of unique and shared skills, and encourage teamwork; pandemic and emergency preparedness and response (including in fragile and humanitarian settings); and principles of respectful care.

of the health workforce and its work environment; leadership and governance; and service delivery. These investments should be considered at country, regional and global levels by governments, policy-makers, regulatory authorities, education institutions, professional associations, international organizations, global partnerships, donor agencies, civil society organizations and researchers. Within several of these areas, there are ongoing efforts to build on, including frameworks, mechanisms and tools for strengthening midwifery *(34, 150)* and for assessment and accreditation of midwifery education *(51, 63, 151)*, including an action plan to strengthen quality midwifery education *(51)*.

INVEST IN

 Midwife-led improvements to SRMNAH service delivery

Communications and partnerships

- Communicate evidence about the benefits of midwives as key SRMNAH service providers.

- Promote continuous partnership between midwives and service users to build trust, communication and mutual respect. Seek out, listen to and act on service users' voices as part of this process.

- Treat midwives as equal and respected partners at local, national, regional and global levels.

Midwife-led models of care

- Develop a conducive and enabling environment in which midwife-led continuity of care can flourish, including collaborative partnerships with other health-care professionals such as nurses, obstetricians, gynaecologists, anaesthetists, paediatricians and neonatologists.

Optimized roles for midwives

- Recognize the potential of midwives to contribute to a wide range of SRMNAH services and initiatives in addition to maternity care (e.g. addressing sexual and reproductive health and rights and promoting self-care interventions).

- Prepare and enable midwives to meet the needs of user groups at risk of discrimination due to characteristics such as age, disability, gender identity, sexual orientation, race and religion.

- Prepare and enable midwives to participate in audit and data collection processes, including Maternal and Perinatal Death Surveillance and Response.

Applying the lessons from Covid-19

- Apply the lessons learned from Covid-19 to build resilience to future health shocks so they do not negatively impact SRMNAH worker education, service delivery and the enabling work environment.

INVEST IN

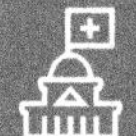 Midwifery leadership and governance

- Create positions at national and subnational levels, including senior midwives within national ministries of health, so that midwives are in all places where SRMNAH decisions are made.

- Engage midwives in relevant policy decisions, programme planning, implementation and monitoring and evaluation at subnational, national, regional and global levels.

- Build and strengthen institutional capacity for midwives to provide leadership and advocacy which will enable high-quality care and increase engagement in health policy decision-making and planning processes.

New addition to the family,
Sydney, Australia.
© Trinh Mai-Guico.

Midwives' association

The SoWMy research agenda

SoWMy 2021 highlights a number of gaps in knowledge about the SRMNAH workforce, especially midwives, that need further research. A global midwifery research alliance has been established to focus on three research priorities identified in the 2014 Lancet Series on Midwifery: (i) investigate the impact of quality maternal and newborn care and in particular the contribution of midwifery, on maternal, newborn and related outcomes across diverse settings; (ii) identify and describe aspects of care that optimize or disturb physiology for all childbearing women and their fetus/newborn/infant; and (iii) determine which indicators, measures and benchmarks are most valuable in assessing quality maternal and newborn care across settings, including the views of childbearing women; and develop new ones to address identified gaps *(152)*.

In addition to these research priorities, the SoWMy 2021 research agenda includes:

- studying countries with more than one midwife education pathway to understand how graduates from different pathways compare in terms of their competencies, and where and how they are deployed;

- conducting a review of approaches to and progress in equipping the workforce to meet the specific SRMNAH needs of adolescents, a large and important group of service users;

- conducting an in-depth analysis of subnational SRMNAH workforce data;

- exploring the reasons for variations in midwives' scope of practice between countries and regions;

- analysing the specific role of midwives in addressing reductions in morbidity and mortality of women and newborns; and

- evaluating the strengths and weaknesses of approaches used during the Covid-19 pandemic and recommending ways to maintain the continuity of midwifery education and essential midwifery and other SRMNAH services during future pandemics and other public health emergencies.

SoWMy 2021 and its research agenda are intended to support improvements to the availability, accessibility, acceptability and quality of the SRMNAH workforce, in all parts of the world. All stakeholders are encouraged to use it to inform their strategic planning towards 2030 and beyond.

Dedicated SRMNAH equivalent (DSE)*: Headcount adjusted for % of clinical time spent on SRMNAH care, to estimate the amount of health worker clinical time available to deliver SRMNAH interventions.

Demand for SRMNAH workers*: The number of SMRNAH workers that a country's health system can support in terms of funded positions or economic demand for SRMNAH services.

Gender: The characteristics of women, men, girls and boys that are socially constructed. As a social construct, gender varies from society to society, and can also change over time. Gender is hierarchical and produces inequalities that intersect with other social and economic inequalities. Gender interacts with but is different from sex, which refers to the different biological and physiological characteristics of females, males and intersex persons, such as chromosomes, hormones and reproductive organs.[1]

Gender transformation Gender transformation actively examines, questions and changes rigid gender norms and imbalances of power that advantage boys and men over girls and women. It aspires to tackle the root causes of gender inequality and to reshape unequal power relations: it moves beyond individual improvement for girls and women towards redressing the power dynamics and structures that reinforce gendered inequalities.[2]

Leadership role (in relation to midwives)*: "Leadership role" as defined in the ICM survey may refer to a number of management, supervisory and executive titles, including midwives:

- in Ministry of Health positions (e.g. Chief Midwife, midwife advisor, national midwife director, maternity advisory positions)

- leading regional or local maternity facilities (e.g. midwife director, midwife advisor to chief executive or senior team, midwives in charge of maternity units/wards)

- leading professional midwives' associations (e.g. President, Chief Executive/Director)

- leading midwifery regulatory authorities (e.g. Chair of Midwifery Council, Chief Executive/Director)

- leading midwifery education programmes (e.g. Head of Midwifery School, Director of Midwifery, Head of Midwifery Programme).

Midwife: A responsible and accountable professional who works in partnership with women to give the necessary support, care and advice during pregnancy, labour and the postpartum period, to conduct births on the midwife's own responsibility and to provide care for the newborn and the infant. This care includes preventative measures, the promotion of normal birth, the detection of complications in mother and child, the accessing of medical care or other appropriate assistance and the carrying out of emergency measures. The midwife has an important task in health counselling and education, not only for the woman, but also within the family and the community. This work should involve antenatal education and preparation for parenthood and may extend to women's health, sexual or reproductive health and childcare. A midwife may practise in any setting including the home, community, hospitals, clinics or health units.[3]

Midwife-led care: The midwife is the lead health-care professional, responsible for planning, organizing and delivering care.[4]

Midwife-led continuity of care: Midwife-led continuity of care models, in which a known midwife, or a small group of known midwives, supports a woman throughout the antenatal, childbirth and postnatal continuum, are recommended for pregnant women in settings with well functioning midwifery programmes.[5]

Need for SRMNAH workers*: The amount of SRMNAH worker time needed to achieve universal coverage of the essential SRMNAH interventions listed in the Global Strategy for Women's, Children's and Adolescents' Health.

Nurse: A person who has successfully completed a programme of basic, generalized nursing education and is authorized by the appropriate regulatory authority to practise nursing. Basic nursing education is a formally recognized programme of study providing a broad and sound foundation in the behavioural, life and nursing sciences for the general practice of nursing, for a leadership role, and for post-basic education for specialty or advanced nursing practice. The nurse is prepared and authorized (i) to engage in the general scope of nursing practice, including the promotion of health, prevention of illness, and care of physically ill, mentally ill and disabled people of all ages and in all health-care and other community settings; (ii) to carry out health-care teaching; (iii) to participate fully as a member of the health-care team; (iv) to supervise and train nursing and health-care auxiliaries; and (v) to be involved in research.[6]

Nurse-midwife*: In National Health Workforce Accounts, countries reported how many of their professional and association professional nurses had "midwifery training", defined as having "successfully completed a midwifery education programme and acquired the requisite qualifications to be registered and/or legally licensed to practise as a midwife". In SoWMy 2021, these "nurses with midwifery training" are referred to as "nurse-midwives", but it is recognized that not all countries use this terminology and that those in the "nurse-midwives" category are not necessarily all engaged in providing midwifery care.

Nursing workforce excluding those with midwifery training*: All persons with a nursing qualification (professional or associate professional) with the exception of nurse professionals or nurse associate professionals with midwifery training who are counted as part of the "wider midwifery workforce" and subtracted from the overall nursing workforce.

Percentage met demand (PMD)*: The number of "dedicated SRMNAH equivalent" (DSE) workers projected in 2030 as a percentage of the number of DSE workers that a country is projected to be able to afford to employ in 2030.

Potential met need (PMN)*: The percentage of health worker time needed for universal coverage of essential SRMNAH interventions that could be delivered by the current workforce if it was educated to global standards, equitably distributed and working within an enabling environment.

Sexual, reproductive, maternal, newborn and adolescent health (SRMNAH) care: The continuum of sexual and reproductive health care and maternal and newborn health care, including for adolescents. Sexual health care involves the enhancement of life and personal relationships, not merely counselling and care related to procreation and sexually transmitted infections. Reproductive health enables people to have a responsible, satisfying and safe sex life, to have children, and to decide if, when and how often to do so.[7]

SRMNAH doctors*: Generalist medical practitioners, obstetricians, gynaecologists and paediatricians.

Supply of health workers: The number of health workers available to provide clinical services.

Wider midwifery workforce*: All persons who have successfully completed a midwifery education programme, whether they are midwives (professionals or associate professionals) or nurses (professional or associate professional) with midwifery training. Completion of such an education programme does not necessarily mean that someone meets the above definition of a midwife. Nurses with midwifery training have been subtracted from the nursing workforce for the purposes of this report.

* This term is specific to SoWMy 2021: it is not standard terminology

GLOSSARY REFERENCES

1. Gender and health. Geneva: World Health Organization; 2021 (https://www.who.int/health-topics/gender#tab=tab_1, accessed 3 March 2021).

2. Technical note on gender-transformative approaches in the global programme to end child marriage phase II: a summary for practitioners. New York: United Nations Children's Fund; 2019 (https://www.unicef.org/media/58196/file, accessed 8 February 2021).

3. International definition of the midwife. The Hague: International Confederation of Midwives; 2017 (https://www.internationalmidwives.org/assets/files/definitions-files/2018/06/eng-definition_of_the_midwife-2017.pdf, accessed 8 February 2021).

4. Position statement: midwifery led care, the first choice for all women. The Hague: International Confederation of Midwives; 2017 (https://www.internationalmidwives.org/assets/files/statement-files/2018/04/eng-midwifery-led-care-the-first-choice-for-all-women.pdf, accessed 16 February 2021).

5. WHO recommendations: intrapartum care for a positive childbirth experience. Geneva: World Health Organization; 2018 (https://www.who.int/reproductivehealth/publications/intrapartum-care-guidelines/en/, accessed 9 March 2021).

6. Definition of a nurse. Geneva: International Council of Nurses; 1987 (https://www.icn.ch/nursing-policy/nursing-definitions, accessed 20 February 2021).

7. Sexual and reproductive health. Geneva: World Health Organization; 2021 (https://www.euro.who.int/en/health-topics/Life-stages/sexual-and-reproductive-health/sexual-and-reproductive-health, accessed 8 February 2021).

REFERENCES

1. Protect the progress: rise, refocus and recover. 2020 progress report on the Every Woman Every Child strategy for women's, children's and adolescents' health (2016–2030). Geneva: World Health Organization and United Nations Children's Fund; 2020 (https://apps.who.int/iris/handle/10665/336219, accessed 8 March 2021).

2. World Health Organization, United Nations Children's Fund, United Nations Population Fund, World Bank Group, United Nations Population Division. Maternal mortality: levels and trends 2000 to 2017. Geneva: World Health Organization; 2019 (https://www.who.int/reproductivehealth/publications/maternal-mortality-2000-2017/en/, accessed 8 March 2021).

3. United Nations Inter-agency Group for Child Mortality Estimation. A neglected tragedy: the global burden of stillbirths. New York: United Nations Children's Fund; 2020 (https://www.unicef.org/reports/neglected-tragedy-global-burden-of-stillbirths-2020, accessed 8 March 2021).

4. United Nations Inter-agency Group for Child Mortality Estimation. Levels and trends in child mortality: 2020 report. New York: United Nations Children's Fund; 2020 (https://www.un.org/development/desa/pd/sites/www.un.org.development.desa.pd/files/unpd_2020_levels-and-trends-in-child-mortality-igme-.pdf, accessed 8 March 2021).

5. Global delivery care coverage and trends 2014–2019. New York: United Nations Children's Fund; 2020 (https://data.unicef.org/topic/maternal-health/delivery-care/, accessed 12 February 2021).

6. Family planning. New York: United Nations Population Fund; 2021 (https://www.unfpa.org/family-planning, accessed 30 April 2021).

7. Sully E, Biddlecom A, Darroch JE, Riley T, Ashford LS, Lince-Deroche N, et al. Adding it up: investing in sexual and reproductive health 2019. New York: The Guttmacher Institute; 2020 (https://www.guttmacher.org/report/adding-it-up-investing-in-sexual-reproductive-health-2019#, accessed 30 April 2021).

8. Endler M, Al-Haidari T, Benedetto C, Chowdhury S, Christilaw J, El Kak F, et al. How the coronavirus disease 2019 pandemic is impacting sexual and reproductive health and rights and response: results from a global survey of providers, researchers, and policy-makers. Acta Obstet Gynecol Scand. 2020. doi: 10.1111/aogs.14043.

9. Every Woman Every Child. The global strategy for women's, children's and adolescents' health 2016–2030. Geneva: World Health Organization; 2015 (https://www.who.int/life-course/partners/global-strategy/global-strategy-2016-2030/en/, accessed 9 March 2021).

10. Transforming our world: the 2030 agenda for sustainable development. New York: United Nations; 2015 (https://sdgs.un.org/sites/default/files/publications/21252030%20Agenda%20for%20Sustainable%20Development%20web.pdf, accessed 17 March 2021).

11. Human rights and the 2030 agenda for sustainable development. Geneva: United Nations Office of the High Commissioner for Human Rights; 2021 (https://www.ohchr.org/en/issues/SDGS/pages/the2030agenda.aspx, accessed 7 February 2021).

12. Global strategy on human resources for health: workforce 2030. Geneva: World Health Organization; 2016 (https://www.who.int/hrh/resources/pub_globstrathrh-2030/en/, accessed 17 March 2021).

13. Oliver K, Parolin Z. Assessing the policy and practice impact of an international policy initiative: the State of the World's Midwifery 2014. BMC Health Serv Res. 2018;18(1):499. doi: 10.1186/s12913-018-3294-4.

14. International standard classification of occupations (ISCO). Geneva: International Labour Organization; 2008 (https://www.ilo.org/public/english/bureau/stat/isco/isco08/index.htm, accessed 6 February 2021).

15. Partnerships between professional midwives and traditional caregivers with midwifery skills. The Hague: International Confederation of Midwives; 2008 (https://www.internationalmidwives.org/assets/files/statement-files/2018/04/eng-partnerships-between-midwives-and-traditional-caregivers.pdf, accessed 15 February 2021).

16. State of the world's nursing. Geneva: World Health Organization; 2020 (https://www.who.int/publications/i/item/9789240003279, accessed 8 March 2021).

17. High-Level Commission on Health Employment and Economic Growth. Working for health and growth: investing in the health workforce. Geneva: World Health Organization; 2016 (https://www.who.int/hrh/com-heeg/reports/en/, accessed 8 March 2021).

18. National health workforce accounts (NHWA). Geneva: World Health Organization; 2021 (https://www.who.int/hrh/statistics/nhwa/en/, accessed 7 February 2021).

19. International Confederation of Midwives, Direct Relief. Global midwives hub. Santa Barbara: Direct Relief; 2021 (https://www.globalmidwiveshub.org/, accessed 15 February 2021).

20. Sexual, reproductive, maternal, newborn, child and adolescent health policy survey 2018–19. Geneva: World Health Organization; 2020 (https://www.who.int/docs/default-source/mca-documents/policy-survey-reports/srmncah-policysurvey2018-fullreport-pt-1.pdf?sfvrsn=930f5059_2, accessed 8 March 2021).

21. Aith F, Castilla Martinez M, Cho M, Dussault G, Harris M, Padilla M, et al. Is COVID-19 a turning point for the health workforce? Rev Panam Salud Publica. 2020;44:e102. doi: 10.26633/RPSP.2020.102.

22. Call to action: COVID-19. Geneva: Partnership for Maternal, Newborn & Child Health; 2020 (https://www.who.int/pmnch/media/news/2020/PMNCH-Call-to-Action-C19.pdf?ua=1, accessed 6 February 2021).

23. United Nations Population Fund, World Health Organization, International Confederation of Midwives. State of the world's midwifery: delivering health, saving lives. New York: United Nations Population Fund; 2011 (https://www.unfpa.org/sites/default/files/pub-pdf/en_SOWMR_Full.pdf, accessed 17 March 2021).

24. United Nations Population Fund, World Health Organization, International Confederation of Midwives. State of the world's midwifery: a universal pathway. A woman's right to health. New York: United Nations Population Fund; 2014 (https://www.unfpa.org/sowmy, accessed 8 March 2021).

25. Nove A, Boyce M. The state of the Pacific's reproductive, maternal, newborn, child and adolescent health workforce. Suva: United Nations Population Fund Pacific Sub-Regional Office; 2019 (https://pacific.unfpa.org/en/publications/state-pacifics-rmncah-workforce-2019-report, accessed 8 March 2021).

26. Nove A, Boyce M, Michel-Schuldt M. Analysis of the sexual, reproductive, maternal, newborn and adolescent health workforce in East and Southern Africa. Johannesburg: United Nations Population Fund East and Southern Africa Regional Office; 2017 (https://esaro.unfpa.org/en/publications/state-worlds-midwifery-analysis-sexual-reproductive-maternal-newborn-and-adolescent, accessed 8 March 2021).

27. Nove A, Guerra-Arias M, Pozo-Martin P, Homer C, Matthews Z. Analysis of the midwifery workforce in selected Arab countries. Cairo: United Nations Population Fund Arab States Regional Office; 2015 (https://arabstates.unfpa.org/en/publications/analysis-midwifery-workforce-selected-arab-countries, accessed 22 March 2021).

28. Camacho AV, Land S, Thompson JE. Strengthening midwifery in Latin America and the Caribbean: a report on the collaboration between the Regional Office for Latin America and the Caribbean of the United Nations Population Fund and the International Confederation of Midwives, 2011–2014. Panama City: Regional Office for Latin America and the Caribbean of the United Nations Population Fund; 2014.

29. Kanem N. Midwives – defenders of women's rights. Bangkok: United Nations Population Fund; 2019 (https://asiapacific.unfpa.org/en/news/midwives%E2%80%94-defenders-womens-rights#:~:text=Midwives%20are%20public%20health%20heroes,the%20most%20basic%20human%20rights, accessed 6 February 2021).

30. Nove A, Friberg IK, de Bernis L, McConville F, Moran AC, Najjemba M, et al. Potential impact of midwives in preventing and reducing maternal and neonatal mortality and stillbirths: a Lives Saved Tool modelling study. Lancet Glob Health. 2021;9(1):e24–e32. doi: 10.1016/S2214-109X(20)30397-1.

31. Sandall J, Soltani H, Gates S, Shennan A, Devane D. Midwife-led continuity models versus other models of care for childbearing women. Cochrane Database Syst Rev. 2016(4):CD004667. doi: 10.1002/14651858.CD004667.pub5.

32. Chapman A, Nagle C, Bick D, Lindberg R, Kent B, Calache J, et al. Maternity service organisational interventions that aim to reduce caesarean section: a systematic review and meta-analysis. BMC Pregnancy Childbirth. 2019;19(1):206. doi: 10.1186/s12884-019-2351-2.

33. Renfrew MJ, McFadden A, Bastos MH, Campbell J, Channon AA, Cheung NF, et al. Midwifery and quality care: findings from a new evidence-informed framework for maternal and newborn care. Lancet. 2014;384(9948):1129–45. doi: 10.1016/S0140-6736(14)60789-3.

34. Nove A, Hoope-Bender PT, Moyo NT, Bokosi M. The midwifery services framework: what is it, and why is it needed? Midwifery. 2018;57:54–8. doi: 10.1016/j.midw.2017.11.003.

35. WHO recommendations: intrapartum care for a positive childbirth experience. Geneva: World Health Organization; 2018 (https://www.who.int/reproductivehealth/publications/intrapartum-care-guidelines/en/, accessed 9 March 2021).

36. Medley N, Vogel JP, Care A, Alfirevic Z. Interventions during pregnancy to prevent preterm birth: an overview of Cochrane systematic reviews. Cochrane Database Syst Rev. 2018;11(11):CD012505. doi: 10.1002/14651858.CD012505.pub2.

37. Tracy SK, Hartz DL, Tracy MB, Allen J, Forti A, Hall B, et al. Caseload midwifery care versus standard maternity care for women of any risk: M@NGO, a randomised controlled trial. Lancet. 2013;382:1723–32. doi: 10.1016/S0140-6736(13)61406-3.

38. Tracy SK, Welsh A, Hall B, Hartz D, Lainchbury A, Bisits A, et al. Caseload midwifery compared to standard or private obstetric care for first time mothers in a public teaching hospital in Australia: a cross sectional study of cost and birth outcomes. BMC Pregnancy Childbirth. 2014;14(46). doi: 10.1186/1471-2393-14-46.

39. Dixon L, Guilliland K, editors. Continuity of midwifery care in Aotearoa New Zealand: partnership in action. Christchurch, New Zealand: New Zealand College of Midwives; 2019 (https://www.midwife.org.nz/midwives/publications/continuity-of-care-in-aotearoa/, accessed 17 March 2021).

40. Guilliland K, Pairman S. The midwifery partnership: a model for practice. Wellington, New Zealand: Department of Nursing and Midwifery, Victoria University of Wellington; 1995.

41. Pairman S. Women-centred midwifery: partnerships or professional friendships? In: Kirkham M, editor. The midwife–mother relationship. London: Macmillan; 2000.

42. Van Lerberghe W, Matthews Z, Achadi E, Ancona C, Campbell J, Channon A, et al. Country experience with strengthening of health systems and deployment of midwives in countries with high maternal mortality. Lancet. 2014;384(9949):1215–25. doi: 10.1016/S0140-6736(14)60919-3.

43. Road map for accelerating the reduction of maternal and neonatal morbidity and mortality in Malawi. Lilongwe: Republic of Malawi Ministry of Health; 2012 (https://www.healthynewbornnetwork.org/hnn-content/uploads/Malawi-Roadmap-for-Reducing-MN-mortality-2012.pdf, accessed 8 March 2021).

44. The DHS Program. STATcompiler. Washington DC: USAID; 2021 (https://www.statcompiler.com/en/, accessed 5 February 2021).

45. Ir P, Korachais C, Chheng K, Horemans D, Van Damme W, Meessen B. Boosting facility deliveries with results-based financing: a mixed-methods evaluation of the government midwifery incentive scheme in Cambodia. BMC Pregnancy Childbirth. 2015;15:170. doi: 10.1186/s12884-015-0589-x.

46. Cronie DJ. Hospital midwives: an examination of the role, diversity and practice conditions of Dutch hospital midwives. Maastricht: Maastricht University; 2019. doi: 10.26481/dis.20191003dc.

47. Waelput AJM, Sijpkens MK, Lagendijk J, van Minde MRC, Raat H, Ernst-Smelt HE, et al. Geographical differences in perinatal health and child welfare in the Netherlands: rationale for the healthy pregnancy 4 all–2 program. BMC Pregnancy Childbirth. 2017;17(1):254. doi: 10.1186/s12884-017-1425-2.

48. Kansrijke Start. Amsterdam: Ministerie van Volksgezondheid Welzijn en Sport; 2018 (https://www.kansrijkestartnl.nl/, accessed 13 March 2021).

49. Hingstman L, Kenens R. Cijfers uit de registratie van verloskundigen. Peiling 2008. Utrecht: Nivel; 2009 (https://www.nivel.nl/nl/publicatie/cijfers-uit-de-registratie-van-verloskundigen-peiling-2008, accessed 17 March 2021).

50. Gavine A, MacGillivray S, McConville F, Gandhi M, Renfrew MJ. Pre-service and in-service education and training for maternal and newborn care providers in low- and middle-income countries: an evidence review and gap analysis. Midwifery. 2019;78:104–13. doi: 10.1016/j.midw.2019.08.007.

51. World Health Organization, United Nations Population Fund, United Nations Children's Fund, International Confederation of Midwives. Strengthening quality midwifery education for universal health coverage 2030: framework for action. Geneva: World Health Organization; 2019 (https://www.who.int/maternal_child_adolescent/topics/quality-of-care/midwifery/strengthening-midwifery-education/en/, accessed 8 March 2021).

52. Graf J, Simoes E, Blaschke S, Plappert CF, Hill J, Riefert MJ, et al. Academisation of the midwifery profession and the implementation of higher education in the context of the new requirements for licensure. Geburtshilfe Frauenheilkd. 2020;80(10):1008–15. doi: 10.1055/a-1138-1948.

53. Bogren M, Banu A, Parvin S, Chowdhury M, Erlandsson K. Findings from a context specific accreditation assessment at 38 public midwifery education institutions in Bangladesh. Women Birth. 2021;34(1):e76–e83. doi: 10.1016/j.wombi.2020.06.009.

54. Ahmadi G, Shahriari M, Keyvanara M, Kohan S. Midwifery students' experiences of learning clinical skills in Iran: a qualitative study. Int J Med Educ. 2018;9:64–71. doi: 10.5116/ijme.5a88.0344.

55. Homer CSE, Turkmani S, Rumsey M. The state of midwifery in small island Pacific nations. Women Birth. 2017;30(3):193–9. doi: 10.1016/j.wombi.2017.02.012.

56. Homer CSE, Castro Lopes S, Nove A, Michel-Schuldt M, McConville F, Moyo NT, et al. Barriers to and strategies for addressing the availability, accessibility, acceptability and quality of the sexual, reproductive, maternal, newborn and adolescent health workforce: addressing the post-2015 agenda. BMC Pregnancy Childbirth. 2018;18(1):55. doi: 10.1186/s12884-018-1686-4.

57. Filby A, McConville F, Anayda P. What prevents quality midwifery care? A systematic mapping of barriers in low- and middle-income countries from the provider perspective. PLoS ONE. 2016;11(5):e0153391. doi: 10.1371/journal.pone.0153391.

58. Strengthening quality midwifery education: meeting report, July 25–26 2016. Geneva: World Health Organization; 2016 (https://apps.who.int/iris/bitstream/handle/10665/259278/WHO-FWC-MCA-17.12-eng.pdf?sequence=1, accessed 17 March 2021).

59. McFadden A, Gupta S, Marshall JL, Shinwell S, Sharma B, McConville F, et al. Systematic review of barriers to, and facilitators of, the provision of high-quality midwifery services in India. Birth. 2020;47(4):304–21. doi: 10.1111/birt.12498.

60. Regional offices. Geneva: World Health Organization; 2021 (https://www.who.int/about/who-we-are/regional-offices, accessed 2 April 2021).

61. World Bank country and lending groups. Washington DC: World Bank; 2021 (https://datahelpdesk.worldbank.org/knowledgebase/articles/906519-world-bank-country-and-lending-groups, accessed 2 April 2021).

62. Nove A, Pairman S, Bohle LF, Garg S, Moyo NT, Michel-Schuldt M, et al. The development of a global midwifery education accreditation programme. Glob Health Action. 2018;11(1):1489604. doi: 10.1080/16549716.2018.1489604.

63. Midwifery education accreditation programme (MEAP). The Hague: International Confederation of Midwives; 2021 (https://www.internationalmidwives.org/icm-publications/meap.html, accessed 7 March 2021).

64. Bogren M, Kaboru BB, Berg M. Barriers to delivering quality midwifery education programmes in the Democratic Republic of Congo – an interview study with educators and clinical preceptors. Women Birth. 2021;34(1):e67–e75. doi: 10.1016/j.wombi.2020.06.004.

65. Bogren MU, Wiseman A, Berg M. Midwifery education, regulation and association in six South Asian countries – a descriptive report. Sex Reprod Healthc. 2012;3(2):67–72. doi: 10.1016/j.srhc.2012.03.004.

66. Task sharing to improve access to family planning/contraception. Geneva: World Health Organization; 2017 (https://www.who.int/reproductivehealth/publications/task-sharing-access-fp-contraception/en/, accessed 30 January 2021).

67. Furuta M. 2020 international year of midwifery – in the midst of a pandemic. Midwifery. 2020;87:102739. doi: 10.1016/j.midw.2020.102739.

68. COVID-19 advice for students and educators. Canberra City: Australian College of Midwives; 2021 (https://www.midwives.org.au/covid-19-advice-students-and-educators, accessed 1 February 2021).

69. Morin KH. Nursing education after COVID-19: same or different? J Clin Nurs. 2020;29(17-18):3117–9. doi: 10.1111/jocn.15322.

70. Luyben A, Fleming V, Vermeulen J. Midwifery education in COVID-19-time: challenges and opportunities. Midwifery. 2020;89:102776. doi: 10.1016/j.midw.2020.102776.

71. NMC statement: enabling student education and supporting the workforce. London: Nursing and Midwifery Council; 2021 (https://www.nmc.org.uk/news/news-and-updates/statement-enabling-student-education-and-supporting-the-workforce/, accessed 1 February 2021).

72. Renfrew MJ, Bradshaw G, Burnett A, Byrom A, Entwistle F, King K, et al. Sustaining quality education and practice learning in a pandemic and beyond: 'I have never learnt as much in my life, as quickly, ever'. Midwifery. 2021;94:102915. doi: 10.1016/j.midw.2020.102915.

73. Midwives during COVID-19 – a position statement from the professional midwives associations of Latin America. The Hague: International Confederation of Midwives; 2020 (https://internationalmidwives.org/icm-news/midwives-during-covid-19-a-position-statement-from-the-professional-midwives-associations-of-latin-america.html, accessed 10 February 2021).

74. Promoción de salud mujer y RN / obstetricia UChile. Santiago: University of Chile; 2021 (https://www.youtube.com/channel/UCW8wGp1N58bf_DIdDss4ioQ, accessed 10 February 2021).

75. Recursos de interés. Santiago: University of Chile; 2021 (http://deptopromomujeryrn.med.uchile.cl/wp/, accessed 10 February 2021).

76. Respositorio UNFPA. Santiago: University of Chile; 2021 (http://depto-promomujeryrn.med.uchile.cl/wp/repositorio-unfpa/, accessed 10 February 2021).

77. Covid-19 educational materials. Couva, Trinidad: Caribbean Regional Midwives Association; 2021 (https://caribbean-regionalmidwivesassociation.com/covid-19-pandemic/, accessed 10 February 2021).

78. Hobbs AJ, Moller AB, Kachikis A, Carvajal-Aguirre L, Say L, Chou D. Scoping review to identify and map the health personnel considered skilled birth attendants in low- and middle-income countries from 2000–2015. PLoS ONE. 2019;14(2):e0211576. doi: 10.1371/journal.pone.0211576.

79. World Health Organization, United Nations Population Fund, United Nations Children's Fund, International Confederation of Midwives, International Council of Nurses, International Federation of Gynecology and Obstetrics, et al. Definition of skilled health personnel providing care during childbirth. Geneva: World Health Organization; 2018 (https://www.who.int/publications/i/item/definition-of-skilled-health-personnel-providing-care-during-childbirth, accessed 6 February 2021).

80. Decade for health workforce strengthening in the South-East Asia Region 2015–2024: second review of progress. Delhi: World Health Organization Regional Office for South-East Asia; 2018 (https://apps.who.int/iris/handle/10665/274310, accessed 9 March 2021).

81. ten Hoope-Bender P, Nove A, Sochas L, Matthews Z, Homer CSE, Pozo-Martin F. The 'dream team' for sexual, reproductive, maternal, newborn and adolescent health: an adjusted service target model to estimate the ideal mix of health care professionals to cover population need. Hum Resour Health. 2017;15:46. doi: 10.1186/s12960-017-0221-4.

82. Langlois ÉV, Miszkurka M, Zunzunegui MV, Ghaffar A, Ziegler D, Karp I. Inequities in postnatal care in low- and middle-income countries: a systematic review and meta-analysis. Bull World Health Organ. 2015;93:259–70. doi: 10.2471/BLT.14.140996.

83. Second round of the national pulse survey on continuity of essential health services during the COVID-19 pandemic: January–March 2021. Geneva: World Health Organization; 2021 (https://www.who.int/teams/integrated-health-services/monitoring-health-services/national-pulse-survey-on-continuity-of-essential-health-services-during-the-covid-19-pandemic, accessed 26 April 2021).

84. Sharma KA, Zangmo R, Kumari A, Roy KK, Bharti J. Family planning and abortion services in COVID 19 pandemic. Taiwan J Obstet Gynecol. 2020;59(6):808–11. doi: 10.1016/j.tjog.2020.09.005.

85. Health workforce policy and management in the context of the COVID-19 pandemic response: interim guidance. Geneva: World Health Organization; 2020 (https://apps.who.int/iris/bitstream/handle/10665/337333/WHO-2019-nCoV-health_workforce-2020.1-eng.pdf?sequence=1&isAllowed=y, accessed 17 March 2021).

86. Keep health workers safe to keep patients safe. Geneva: World Health Organization; 2020 (https://www.who.int/news/item/17-09-2020-keep-health-workers-safe-to-keep-patients-safe-who, accessed 5 February 2021).

87. Nguyen LH, Drew DA, Graham MS, Joshi AD, Guo C-G, Ma W, et al. Risk of COVID-19 among front-line health-care workers and the general community: a prospective cohort study. Lancet Public Health. 2020;5(9):e475–e83. doi: https://doi.org/10.1016/S2468-2667(20)30164-X.

88. COVID-19: health worker death toll rises to at least 17000 as organizations call for rapid vaccine rollout. London: Amnesty International; 2021 (https://www.amnesty.org/en/latest/news/2021/03/covid19-health-worker-death-toll-rises-to-at-least-17000-as-organizations-call-for-rapid-vaccine-rollout/?utm_source=TWITTER-IS&utm_medium=social&utm_content=4546684499&utm_campaign=Other&utm_term=Making_the_Case_for_Human_Rights-No, accessed 13 March 2021).

89. Lapor Covid-19. Jakarta: Digital Center for Indonesian Health Workers; 2021 (https://nakes.laporcovid19.org/, accessed 6 February 2021).

90. International Council of Nurses: COVID-19 update, 13 January 2021. Geneva: International Council of Nurses; 2021 (https://www.icn.ch/sites/default/files/inline-files/ICN%20COVID19%20update%20report%20FINAL.pdf, accessed 6 February 2021).

91. McKay D, Heisler M, Mishori R, Catton H, Kloiber O. Attacks against health-care personnel must stop, especially as the world fights COVID-19. Lancet. 2020;395(10239):1743–5. doi: 10.1016/S0140-6736(20)31191-0.

92. Global call to action: protecting midwives to sustain care for women, newborns and their families in the COVID-19 pandemic. The Hague: International Confederation of Midwives; 2020 (https://www.internationalmidwives.org/assets/files/news-files/2020/05/1call-to-action.pdf, accessed 13 February 2021).

93. Bourgeault IL, Maier CB, Dieleman M, Ball J, Mackenzie A, Nancarrow S, et al. The COVID-19 pandemic presents an opportunity to develop more sustainable health workforces. Hum Resour Health. 2020;18:83. doi: 10.1186/s12960-020-00529-0.

94. Castro Lopes S, Guerra-Arias M, Buchan J, Pozo-Martin F, Nove A. A rapid review of the rate of attrition from the health workforce. Hum Resour Health. 2017;15(1):21. doi: 10.1186/s12960-017-0195-2.

95. Liu JX, Goryakin Y, Maeda A, Bruckner T, Scheffler R. Global health workforce labor market projections for 2030. Hum Resour Health. 2017;15(1):11. doi: 10.1186/s12960-017-0187-2.

96. Rehnström Loi U, Gemzell-Danielsson K, Faxelid E, Klingberg-Allvin M. Health care providers' perceptions of and attitudes towards induced abortions in sub-Saharan Africa and Southeast Asia: a systematic literature review of qualitative and quantitative data. BMC Public Health. 2015;15:139. doi: 10.1186/s12889-015-1502-2.

97. Haddad LB, Nour NM. Unsafe abortion: unnecessary maternal mortality. Rev Obstet Gynecol. 2009;2(2):122–6. (https://www.ncbi.nlm.nih.gov/pubmed/19609407, accessed 17 March 2021).

98. Buchan J, Couper ID, Tangcharoensathien V, Thepannya K, Jaskiewicz W, Perfilieva G, et al. Early implementation of WHO recommendations for the retention of health workers in remote and rural areas. Bull World Health Organ. 2013;91(11):834–40. doi: 10.2471/BLT.13.119008.

99. Increasing access to health workers in remote and rural areas through improved retention: global policy recommendations. Geneva: World Health Organization; 2010 (https://www.who.int/hrh/retention/guidelines/en/, accessed 8 March 2021).

100. Matthews Z, Rawlins B, Duong J, Molla YB, Moran AC, Singh K, et al. Geospatial analysis for reproductive, maternal, newborn, child and adolescent health: gaps and opportunities. BMJ Glob Health. 2019;4(Suppl 5):e001702. doi: 10.1136/bmjgh-2019-001702.

101. WorldPop, University of Louisville, Université de Namur, Columbia University. Global high resolution population denominators project. Southampton, UK: WorldPop; 2018 (https://www.worldpop.org/doi/10.5258/SOTON/WP00646, accessed 4 February 2021).

102. WorldPop (University of Southampton School of Geography and Environmental Science). Ghana 1km births. Version 2.0 2015 estimates of numbers of live births per grid square, with national totals adjusted to match UN national estimates on numbers of live births. Southampton, UK: WorldPop; 2017.

103. WorldPop (University of Southampton School of Geography and Environmental Science). Ghana 1km pregnancies. Version 2.0 2015 estimates of numbers of pregnancies per grid square, with national totals adjusted to match national estimates on numbers of pregnancies made by the Guttmacher Institute. Southampton, UK: WorldPop; 2017.

104. Ghana demographic and health survey 2014. Rockville: Ghana Statistical Service, Ghana Health Service and ICF International; 2015 (https://dhsprogram.com/pubs/pdf/FR307/FR307.pdf, accessed 17 March 2021).

105. Bohren MA, Hunter EC, Munthe-Kaas HM, Souza JP, Vogel JP, Gulmezoglu AM. Facilitators and barriers to facility-based delivery in low- and middle-income countries: a qualitative evidence synthesis. Reprod Health. 2014;11(1):71. doi: 10.1186/1742-4755-11-71.

106. Hartz DL, Blain J, Caplice S, Allende T, Anderson S, Hall B, et al. Evaluation of an Australian Aboriginal model of maternity care: The Malabar Community Midwifery Link Service. Women Birth. 2019;32(5):427–36. doi: 10.1016/j.wombi.2019.07.002.

107. Proujansky A. The black midwives changing care for women of color – photo essay. The Guardian. 25 July 2019 (https://www.theguardian.com/society/2019/jul/24/black-midwives-photo-essay, accessed 9 March 2021).

108. Shakibazadeh E, Namadian M, Bohren MA, Vogel JP, Rashidian A, Noguiera Pileggi V, et al. Respectful care during childbirth in health facilities globally: a qualitative evidence synthesis. BJOG. 2017;125(8):932–42. doi: 10.1111/1471-0528.15015.

109. Respectful maternity care charter, 2018 update. Washington DC: White Ribbon Alliance; 2018 (https://www.whiteribbonalliance.org/respectful-maternity-care-charter/, accessed 12 February 2021).

110. Bohren MA, Vogel JP, Tuncalp O, Fawole B, Titiloye MA, Olutayo AO, et al. "By slapping their laps, the patient will know that you truly care for her": A qualitative study on social norms and acceptability of the mistreatment of women during childbirth in Abuja, Nigeria. SSM Popul Health. 2016;2:640–55. doi: 10.1016/j.ssmph.2016.07.003.

111. Sen G, Reddy B, Iyer A. Beyond measurement: the drivers of disrespect and abuse in obstetric care. Reprod Health Matters. 2018;26(53):6–18. doi: 10.1080/09688080.2018.1508173.

112. Bohren MA, Vogel JP, Hunter EC, Lutsiv O, Makh SK, Souza JP, et al. The mistreatment of women during childbirth in health facilities globally: a mixed-methods systematic review. PLoS Med. 2015;12(6). doi: 10.1371/journal.pmed.1001847.

113. Jolivet RR, Warren CE, Sripad P, Ateva E, Gausman J, Mitchell K, et al. Upholding rights under COVID-19: the respectful maternity care charter. Health Hum Rights. 2020;22(1):391–4. (https://www.ncbi.nlm.nih.gov/pmc/articles/PMC7348430/pdf/hhr-22-01-391.pdf, accessed 17 March 2021).

114. Maintaining essential health services: operational guidance for the COVID-19 context interim guidance, 1 June 2020. Geneva: World Health Organization; 2020 (https://www.who.int/publications/i/item/WHO-2019-nCoV-essential-health-services-2020.1, accessed 17 March 2021).

115. What women want! Washington DC: White Ribbon Alliance; 2021 (https://www.whiteribbonalliance.org/whatwomenwant/, accessed 12 February 2021).

116. Pate MA. Why protecting, promoting essential services for women and children is now more critical than ever. World Bank Blogs, 16 October 2020. (https://blogs.worldbank.org/health/why-protecting-promoting-essential-services-women-and-children-now-more-critical-ever, accessed 6 February 2021).

117. Roberton T, Carter ED, Chou VB, Stegmuller AR, Jackson BD, Tam Y, et al. Early estimates of the indirect effects of the COVID-19 pandemic on maternal and child mortality in low-income and middle-income countries: a modelling study. Lancet Glob Health. 2020;8(7):e901–e8. doi: 10.1016/S2214-109X(20)30229-1.

118. Cousins S. COVID-19 has "devastating" effect on women and girls. Lancet. 2020;396(10247):301–2. doi: 10.1016/S0140-6736(20)31679-2.

119. Protecting essential services for women, children and adolescents during COVID-19. Washington DC: The World Bank Group; (https://www.globalfinancingfacility.org/sites/gff_new/files/documents/GFF-IG11-3-Protecting-Essential-Services-in-Times-of-COVID19.pdf, accessed 30 April 2021).

120. Liu Q, Luo D, Haase JE, Gou Q, Wang XQ, Liu S, et al. The experiences of health-care providers during the COVID-19 crisis in China: a qualitative study. Lancet Glob Health. 2020;8(6):e790–8. doi: 10.1016/S2214-109X(20)30204-7.

121. Morgantini LA, Naha U, Wang H, Francavilla S, Acar Ö, Flores JM, et al. Factors contributing to healthcare professional burnout during the COVID-19 pandemic: a rapid turnaround global survey. PLoS ONE. 2020;15(9):e0238217. doi: 10.1371/journal.pone.0238217.

122. Semaan A, Audet C, Huysmans E, Afolabi B, Assarag B, Banke-Thomas A, et al. Voices from the frontline: findings from a thematic analysis of a rapid online global survey of maternal and newborn health professionals facing the COVID-19 pandemic. BMJ Glob Health. 2020;5(6):e002967. doi: 10.1136/bmjgh-2020-002967.

123. Pallangyo E, Nakate MG, Maina R, Fleming V. The impact of Covid-19 on midwives' practice in Kenya, Uganda and Tanzania: a reflective account. Midwifery. 2020;89:102775. doi: 10.1016/j.midw.2020.102775.

124. Analysing and using routine data to monitor the effects of COVID-19 on essential health services: practical guide for national and sub-national decision-makers. Geneva: World Health Organization; 2021 (https://www.who.int/publications/i/item/WHO-2019-nCoV-essential_health_services-monitoring-2021.1, accessed 9 March 2021).

125. Boniol M, McIsaac M, Xu L, Wuliji T, Diallo K, Campbell J. Gender equity in the health workforce: analysis of 104 countries. Health Workforce Working Paper 1. Geneva: World Health Organization; 2019 (https://apps.who.int/iris/bitstream/handle/10665/311314/WHO-HIS-HWF-Gender-WP1-2019.1-eng.pdf?ua=1, accessed 17 March 2021).

126. Magar V, Gerecke M, Dhillon IS, Campbell J. Women's contributions to sustainable development through work in health: using a gender lens to advance a transformative 2030 agenda. In: Buchan J, Dhillon IS, Campbell J, editors. Health Employment and Economic Growth: An Evidence Base. Geneva: World Health Organization; 2017 (https://www.who.int/hrh/resources/WHO-HLC-Report_web.pdf?ua=1, accessed 17 March 2021).

127. Buchan J, Dhillon IS, Campbell J, editors. Health employment and economic growth: an evidence base. Geneva: World Health Organization; 2017 (https://www.who.int/hrh/resources/WHO-HLC-Report_web.pdf?ua=1, accessed 17 March 2021).

128. Delivered by women, led by men: a gender and equity analysis of the global health and social workforce. Geneva: World Health Organization Global Health Workforce Network's Gender Equity Hub; 2019 (https://www.who.int/hrh/resources/health-observer24/en/, accessed 9 March 2021).

129. International Confederation of Midwives, World Health Organization, White Ribbon Alliance. Midwives' voices, midwives' realities: findings from a global consultation on providing quality midwifery care. Geneva: World Health Organization; 2016 (https://apps.who.int/iris/bitstream/handle/10665/250376/9789241510547-eng.pdf, accessed 17 March 2021).

130. ILO violence and harassment convention, 2019 (no.190): 12 ways it can support the COVID-19 response and recovery. Geneva: International Labour Organization; 2020 (https://www.ilo.org/wcmsp5/groups/public/---arabstates/---ro-beirut/documents/briefingnote/wcms_748420.pdf, accessed 10 February 2021).

131. Kang L, Ma S, Chen M, Yang J, Wang Y, Li R, et al. Impact on mental health and perceptions of psychological care among medical and nursing staff in Wuhan during the 2019 novel coronavirus disease outbreak: A cross-sectional study. Brain Behav Immun. 2020;87:11–7. doi: 10.1016/j.bbi.2020.03.028.

132. Theorell T. COVID-19 and working conditions in health care. Psychother Psychosom. 2020;89(4):193–4. doi: 10.1159/000507765.

133. Currie S, Azfar P, Fowler RC. A bold new beginning for midwifery in Afghanistan. Midwifery. 2007;23(3):226–34. doi: 10.1016/j.midw.2007.07.003.

134. Fauveau V, Sherratt DR, de Bernis L. Human resources for maternal health: multi-purpose or specialists? Hum Resour Health. 2008;30(6):21. doi: 10.1186/1478-4491-6-21.

135. Study and work in the EU: set apart by gender. Review of the implementation of the Beijing Platform for Action. Brussels: European Institute for Gender Equality; 2018 (https://eige.europa.eu/publications/study-and-work-eu-set-apart-gender-report, accessed 9 March 2021).

136. George AS, McConville FE, de Vries S, Nigenda G, Sarfraz S, McIsaac M. Violence against female health workers is tip of iceberg of gender power imbalances. BMJ. 2020;371:m3546. doi: 10.1136/bmj.m3546.

137. Improving employment and working conditions in health services. Geneva: International Labour Organization Sectoral Policies Department; 2017 (https://www.ilo.org/sector/activities/sectoral-meetings/WCMS_548288/lang--en/index.htm, accessed 9 March 2021).

138. Jaffré Y, Lange IL. Being a midwife in West Africa: between sensory experiences, moral standards, socio-technical violence and affective constraints. Soc Sci Med. 2021;276:113842. doi: 10.1016/j.socscimed.2021.113842.

139. Eliminating violence and harassment in the world of work. Geneva: International Labour Organization; 2021 (https://www.ilo.org/global/topics/violence-harassment/lang--en/index.htm, accessed 10 February 2021).

140. Note on the proceedings: joint meeting on social dialogue in the health services: institutions, capacity and effectiveness. Geneva: International Labour Organization; 2002 (https://www.ilo.org/public/english/standards/relm/gb/docs/gb286/pdf/jmhs-n.pdf, accessed 6 February 2021).

141. Freedom of association and protection of the right to organise convention. Geneva: International Labour Organization; 1948 (https://www.ilo.org/dyn/normlex/en/f?p=NORMLEXPUB:12100:0::NO::P12100_ILO_CODE:C087, accessed 6 February 2021).

142. DHBs/MERAS multi-employer collective agreement. Auckland: Midwifery Employee Representation and Advisory Services; 2019 (https://meras.midwife.org.nz/wp-content/uploads/sites/4/2019/08/MERAS-MECA-1-February-2018-31-January-2021-Final-signed-version.pdf, accessed 6 February 2021).

143. Sectoral agreement signed between government and MUMN. Valletta, Malta: Malta Union of Midwives and Nurses; 2018 (https://www.mumn.org/news/sectoral-agreement-signed-between-government-and-mumn/, accessed 4 February 2021).

144. Neugründung ver.di-Hebammengruppe Weser-Ems. Berlin: ver.di; 2020 (https://hebammen-niedersachsen.de/verdi-hebammengruppe-weser-ems/, accessed 6 February 2021).

145. ILO nursing personnel convention no. 149: recognize their contribution, address their needs. Geneva: International Labour Organization; 2005 (http://www.ilo.int/sector/Resources/publications/WCMS_508335/lang--en/index.htm, accessed 6 February 2021).

146. Care work and care jobs for the future of decent work. Geneva: International Labour Organization; 2018 (https://www.ilo.org/wcmsp5/groups/public/---dgreports/---dcomm/---publ/documents/publication/wcms_633135.pdf, accessed 17 March 2021).

147. Breen K. Ontario government discriminated against midwives on pay since 2005, human rights tribunal finds. Global News, 25 September 2018. (https://globalnews.ca/news/4484264/ontario-discriminated-against-midwives-pay-equity/, accessed 4 February 2021).

148. Guilliland K, Pittam D. Historic win for midwives. Midwifery News June 2017. Christchurch: New Zealand College of Midwives; 2017 (https://www.midwife.org.nz/wp-content/uploads/2019/02/Pages-from-Midwifery-News-85-June-2017-hi-res.pdf, accessed 5 February 2021).

149. Halonen T, Jilani H, Gilmore K, Bustreo F. Realisation of human rights to health and through health. Lancet. 2017;389(10084):2087–9. doi: 10.1016/S0140-6736(17)31359-4.

150. Strengthening midwifery toolkit. Geneva: World Health Organization; 2011 (https://www.who.int/maternal_child_adolescent/documents/strenthening_midwifery_toolkit/en/, accessed 2 April 2021).

151. Midwifery Assessment Tool for Education (MATE). Geneva: World Health Organization; 2020 (https://www.euro.who.int/en/health-topics/Health-systems/nursing-and-midwifery/publications/2020/midwifery-assessment-tool-for-education-mate-2020, accessed 2 April 2021).

152. Research priorities. Orange, Connecticut: Quality Maternal and Newborn Care Research Alliance; 2021 (https://www.qmnc.org/qmnc-research-alliance/research-priorities/, accessed 2 April 2021).

MIDWIFERY2030
A PATHWAY TO HEALTH

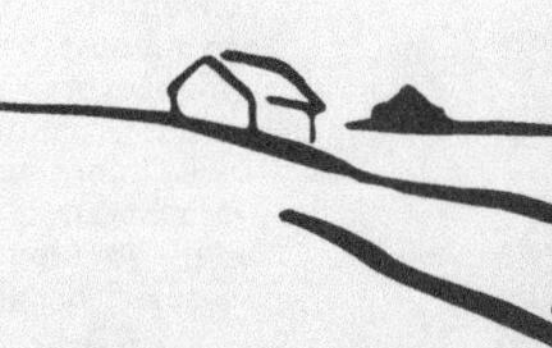

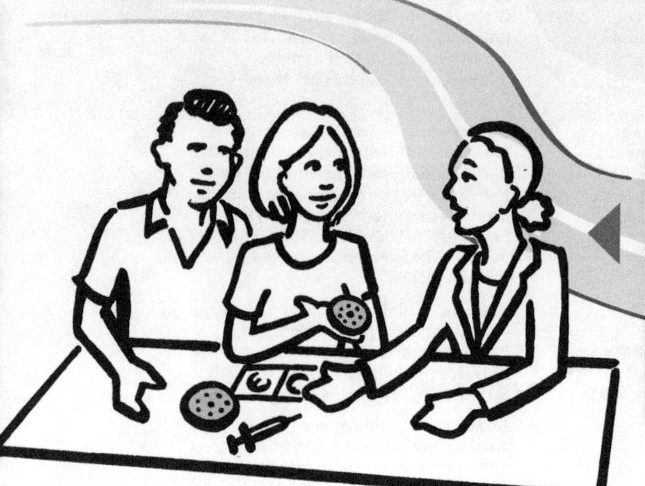

PLANNING AND PREPARING *means:*

- delaying marriage
- completing secondary education
- providing comprehensive sexual education for boys and girls
- protecting yourself against HIV
- maintaining a good health and nutritional status
- planning pregnancies using modern contraceptive methods

ENSURING A HEALTHY START *means:*

- maintaining your health and preparing yourself for pregnancy, childbirth and the early months as a new family
- receiving at least four antenatal care visits, which include discussing birth preparedness and making an emergency plan
- demanding and receiving professional supportive and preventive midwifery care to help you and your baby stay healthy, and to deal with complications effectively, should they arise

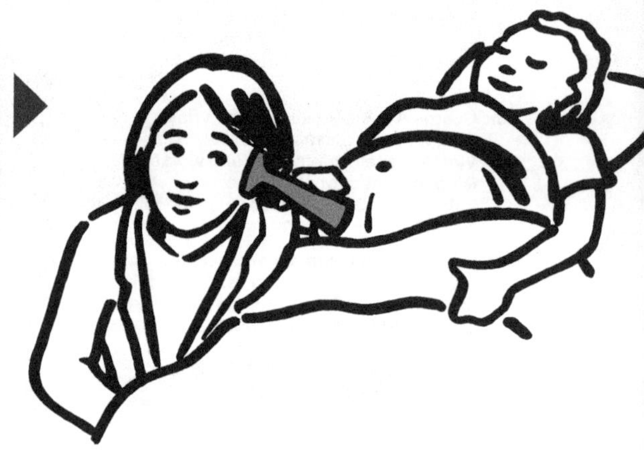

WHAT MAKES THIS POSSIBLE?

1	2	3	4	5
All women of reproductive age, including adolescents, have universal access to midwifery care when needed.	**Governments** provide and are held accountable for a supportive policy environment.	**Governments** and health systems provide and are held accountable for a fully enabled environment.	**Data collection and analysis** are fully embedded in service delivery and development.	**Midwifery care** is prioritized in national health budgets; all women are given universal financial protection.